Beauty Advice

J. Alechno

2010

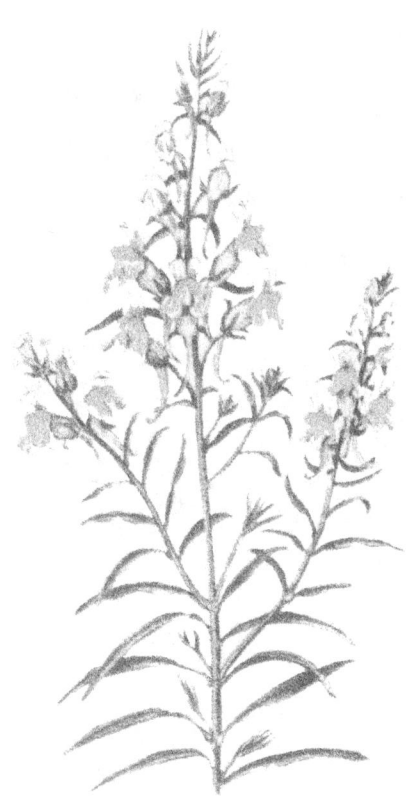

Contents

Foreword

Nowadays when chemistry plays a major role in our lives, words like "natural products" and "natural means" sound very tempting. However, the "natural" skin care products that the market offers us today aren't as natural as they may seem.

Even the most costly skin care products using time-tested recipes for beauty and consisting of vegetable oils and plant extracts only contain tenth or even hundredth parts of natural substances. And as such, the products cannot do without preservatives. In fact, natural oils are quickly oxidized and vegetative emulsifiers present a fine environment for bacteria to thrive in. Many aromatizes, dyes and preservatives have a questionable reputation. Lifeless chemicals will never rejuvenate skin. More so, luxurious skin care products aren't affordable to everyone, not to mention that no one can be sure that they won't cause harmful side effects (allergic reactions, acne, dermatitis, etc.).

But even the use of active vegetable substances in skin care products isn't as efficient as those substances are when remaining inside a plant. In fact, herbs work effectively only due to the connection between biologically active substances and other components. Using natural products correctly can ensure that they never cause harm or any side effects.

For many millennia women have been preserving their beauty and youth using medicinal plants: oils, juices, infusions and extracts of fruits, grasses, berries or nuts. Honey, milk, sour cream, eggs, beeswax and animal fats were widely used for skin care purposes. It is possible to use these recipes within home conditions to prepare creams, ointments, lotions and masks that can improve the health of your skin.

Skin care recipes for normal facial skin

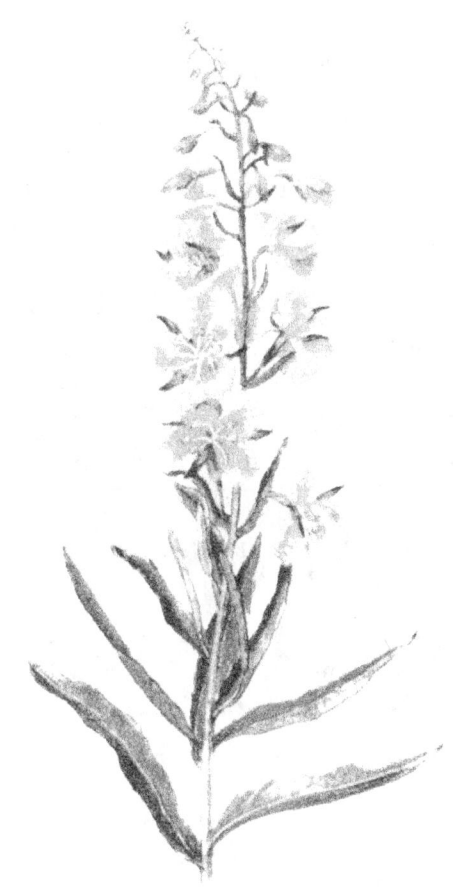

Normal facial skin

Normal skin looks clean and fresh. It has a pink tone (due to even blood supply), remaining ever smooth and elastic. Normal skin contains fair amounts of moisture and grease. It has hardly any visible pores, blackheads or wrinkles. Women with such skin are technically quite lucky, since the normal skin type is extremely rare.

When caring for normal skin, it is important to put effort into preserving its condition for as long as possible. The main thing to remember is to not overly dry the skin. Clean your skin twice a day. After washing, wipe your face with tissues, lotion and a herbal tincture. Lotions possess antiseptic, shrinking and anti-inflammatory properties, toning skin.

Cream moistens skin and protects it from wind, sun and dust. Apply cream to your face in the morning even if you are not going to leave the house. Showering, cooking near a hot stove, etc. - all these actions adversely influence the skin, drying it. Remove surplus cream 10-15 minutes after application with the help of a cosmetic wipe.

In the evening remove makeup, then wash with soap and wipe the skin with lotion followed by an application of nourishing cream.

Apply a nourishing mask once a week. The procedure is done as follows: wash your face, make a compress or vapor bath and then apply a mask.

Normal facial skin cleansing

✓ **Lemon water**

- 1 lemon
- Water

Mix the juice of 1 lemon with about 200 ml of water and leave for one day in a dark cool place. Wipe your skin with the resulting face-wash in the morning.

✓ Poppy water

- 2 tablespoons of poppy seeds
- 200 ml of boiled water

Add 2 tablespoons of poppy seeds to 200 ml of boiled water and let it infuse for one hour. Filter the tincture and wash your face with it.

✓ Cucumber milk

- 1 fresh cucumber
- 200 ml of milk
- 1 teaspoon of olive oil
- 1-2 drops of rose oil

Grate 1 fresh cucumber on a plastic grater, add 200 ml of milk and let it infuse in a closed vessel for one hour. Then filter this mixture, add 1 teaspoon of olive oil, 1-2 drops of rose oil (or 1 teaspoon of rose water) and stir well. This milk can be stored in the refrigerator for three to five days.

✓ Vegetable oil

- Vegetable oil

Dip a cotton wool ball in hot water, wring it out, then moisten it with vegetable oil and wipe the skin on your face and neck. In 1-2 minutes wipe your skin with a cotton wool ball moistened in tea, herbal tincture or boiled water with lemon juice. This procedure clears and moisturizes the skin, making it soft and elastic.

✔ Dandelion oil

- Dried roots and dandelion grass

- Vegetable oil

Crush dried roots and dandelion grass, fill half a glass jar with the crushed material and then fill it with vegetable oil to the brim. Close the jar tightly and leave this mixture for two weeks. Then filter the oil and use for cleansing skin as a substitute for washing, if the skin is inclined to dryness.

✔ Coffee cream-peeling

- Coffee grounds

- Light nourishing cream

To clear and moisten your skin, make a mixture of coffee-grounds and a light nourishing face cream in equal parts. Apply the cream to your skin, massaging it slightly, and wash it off in five to seven minutes.

✔ Bran mask-peeling

- 2 tablespoons of wheat bran

- Water

Mix 2 tablespoons of wheat bran with some water. Rub this mixture into the skin of your face with easy massage movements for two to three minutes. Then wash it off with cool water. Bran clears well, softens and slightly bleaches skin.

✔ Oatmeal mask-peeling

- 2 tablespoons of oatmeal

- Water

Dissolve 2 tablespoons of oatmeal in water until it takes on a gruel-like consistency, and apply it to the skin of your face.

Apply a light massage and wash off the mask with cool water after two to three minutes.

Herbal tinctures and extracts for normal facial skin

✓ Mint-strawberry tincture

- 1 tablespoon of dried peppermint leaves
- 1 tablespoon of wild strawberry leaves
- 250 ml of boiling water

Add 1 tablespoon of dried peppermint leaves and 1 tablespoon of wild strawberry leaves to 250 ml of boiling water and leave for 8-10 hours, filter and store in a refrigerator. Clean your face first and then moisten your skin with this tincture (without rubbing it in).

✓ Rosemary tincture

- 2 teaspoons of rosemary leaves
- 200 ml of boiling water

Add 2 teaspoons of rosemary leaves to 200 ml of boiling water, leave to infuse in a thermos for one hour and filter. Wipe your face with this tincture after washing it. It tones and freshens skin very well.

✓ Flower tincture

- Chamomile flowers
- Linden flowers
- Rose flowers
- 200 ml of boiling water

Mix the chamomile flowers, linden flowers and roses in equal parts and add 2 tablespoons of this mixture to 200 ml of boiling water. Leave to infuse for one hour in a closed pot, then filter and wipe your face with it.

✓ **Dandelion tincture**

- 2 tablespoons of dandelion leaves

- 300 ml of water

Add 2 tablespoons of dandelion leaves to 300 ml of water, heat on a water bath for 15 minutes, let it infuse for 45 minutes at room temperature and then filter. Wipe your face with this tincture in the morning and evening, if your skin is inclined to dryness.

✓ **Linden flowers extract**

- 1-2 tablespoons of linden flowers

- 400 ml of boiling water

Add 1-2 tablespoons of linden flowers to 400 ml of boiling water and boil on a low heat for 5–10 minutes, then filter the cooled extract. Use the extract for washing your face. It does a good job of clearing normal skin inclined to dryness.

Cleansing lotions for normal facial skin

✓ **Yolk-lemon lotion**

- 1 egg yolk

- 30 ml of lemon juice

- 100 ml of vodka

- 50 ml of camphor spirit

Whisk the egg yolk with about 30 ml of lemon juice, add 100 ml of vodka and 50 ml of camphor spirit. Use this lotion for cleansing the skin on your face.

✔ Yolk-honey lotion

- 1 egg yolk
- Half a teaspoon of honey
- 50 ml of vodka
- Camphor spirit
- 75 g of fresh ground almonds

Mix 1 egg yolk with the honey, add about 50 ml of vodka and 25 ml of camphor spirit, add 75 g of fresh ground almonds. This lotion simultaneously clears and nourishes the skin of your face.

✔ Lemon lotion

- 1 lemon juice
- 2 teaspoons of glycerin
- 100 ml of distilled water

Mix the juice of 1 lemon with 2 teaspoons of glycerin and add 100 ml of distilled water. Wipe normal skin inclined to irritation with this lotion.

✔ Lemon-honey lotion

- 1 lemon
- 7 tablespoons of honey
- 2 tablespoons of water

Blend 1 lemon, mix it with 7 tablespoons of honey and keep in a dark place for four days. Then filter this mixture and dilute it with 2 tablespoons of water. Wipe your face with the resulting lotion and wash off with warm water in 15-20 minutes.

✔ Orange lotion

- 1 orange

- 100 ml of vodka

- 1 teaspoon of glycerin

Mince the orange with peel in a mincer, add 100 ml of vodka and leave it to infuse in a closed pan in a dark, cool place for one week. Then filter and add one teaspoon of glycerin. Use this lotion for cleaning your face on a daily basis.

✓ **Cucumber lotion 1**

- 100g of cucumber

- 100 ml of vodka

- 2 teaspoons of glycerin

- 50 ml of water

Grate 100 g of cucumber on a plastic grater, add 100 ml of vodka and leave to infuse for 7-10 days. Then filter this mixture, add 2 teaspoons of glycerin and 50 ml of water. Wipe normal skin with this lotion.

✓ **Cucumber lotion 2**

- Cucumber

- 50 ml of vodka

Grate a fresh cucumber on a plastic grater, wring out 150 ml of juice, mix it with about 50 ml of vodka and leave to infuse for one week. Then filter it and use for cleaning the skin of your face.

✓ **Cucumber lotion 3**

- Cucumber

- 50 ml of tutsan extract

- 25 ml of rose water

Grate a fresh cucumber on a plastic grater, wring out 50 ml of juice and mix it with about 50 ml of tutsan extract and 25 ml of rose water. Store the lotion in a refrigerator. (To prepare a tutsan extract take 1 tablespoon of tutsan herb and add 100 ml of water, then heat on a water bath for 30 minutes, filter and let it cool for 10 minutes.)

✓ Watermelon-peach lotion

- Watermelon juice

- Peach juice

Mix the watermelon juice and peach juice (freshly squeezed juice implied) in equal parts and wipe your face with this mixture. This lotion clears, moistens and nourishes skin well.

✓ Rose lotion

- 2 tablespoons of crushed rose petals

- 200 ml of boiling water

- 1 tablespoon of lemon or orange juice

Add 1 tablespoon of lemon or orange juice to rose petal tincture. Wipe your face with this lotion in the morning and in the evening. (To prepare a rose petal tincture add 2 tablespoons of crushed petals to 200 ml of boiling water and let it infuse in a closed pot at room temperature until it becomes cold.)

✓ Strawberry lotion

- 100 ml of strawberry juice

- 100 ml of vodka

Mix 100 ml of strawberry juice with about 100 ml of vodka and wipe your face with this lotion. If your skin is too sensitive, dilute the lotion with some water. It is possible to freeze strawberry juice and to wipe the skin of your face with an ice cube to freshen and tone it. Wash the juice off with cool water in 15-20 minutes and apply a nourishing cream.

✔ White lily lotion

- White lily flowers

- Vodka

- Distilled water

Fill a dark glass bottle with white lily flowers and pour vodka in to the brim. Leave to infuse in a dark, cool place for 40 days. Then filter it and add distilled water to fill 70% of the bottle's total volume. The lotion can be stored for a long period of time.

✔ Green tea lotion

- 100 g of green tea

- 200 ml of boiling water

- Half a liter of vodka

- Water

Add 100 g of green tea to 200 ml of boiling water and leave to infuse in a closed pot until it becomes cold. Then mix it with half a liter of vodka and leave to infuse - shaking it from time to time - in a dark place for two weeks. Then filter it and dilute with water at a 1:4 proportion. This lotion tones skin and improves complexion.

✔ Herbal lotion

- 1 tablespoon of chamomile flowers

- 1 tablespoon of linden flowers

- 1 tablespoon of mint leaves

- 1 tablespoon of sage grass

- Half a liter of water

- 1 tablespoon of glycerin

Add 1 tablespoon of chamomile flowers, linden blossom, mint leaves and sage grass to half a liter of boiled water, heat on a water bath for 15 minutes, let it infuse for 45 minutes and filter.

Add 1 tablespoon of glycerin to this mixture and wipe your face with it in the morning and in the evening as a substitute for washing it.

Masks for normal facial skin

✔ Sour milk mask

- Almond, olive, sunflower or peach oil

- Kefir, curdled milk or yoghurt

Grease the skin of your face with almond, olive, sunflower or peach oil, then put kefir, curdled milk or yoghurt on it and cover with a damp cotton napkin. Leave the mask on your face for 15-20 minutes. Then wash it off with warm water.

✔ Milk-yeast mask

- 40 g of yeast

- 1 tablespoon of warm milk

Combine 40 g of yeast with 1 tablespoon of warm milk and put 3-4 layers on your face (each layer should be applied as soon as the previous layer dries). Wash the mask off with warm water in 20 minutes. It is recommended that women over 30 years of age apply such masks once or twice a week (the course is comprised of 20 procedures). After the course, skin becomes elastic and smooth.

✔ Yolk-yeast mask

- 25 g of fresh yeast

- Milk

- 1 egg yolk

- 1 teaspoon of honey

- 2 teaspoons of vegetable oil

Combine 25 g of fresh yeast with the milk until it reaches a consistency of sour cream. Mix the egg yolk with 1 teaspoon of honey and then with 2 teaspoons of vegetable oil. Add the diluted yeast and stir well. Put this mixture on your face and leave for 20 minutes. Wash it off with warm water.

✔ Curd mask

- 1 tablespoon of curd

- 1 teaspoon of honey or sour cream

Mix 1 tablespoon of curd with 1 teaspoon of honey or sour cream and put this mixture on your face. Leave the mask for 20 minutes, then remove it with a cotton wool ball moistened in milk. This mask nourishes and moistens skin.

✔ Curd-honey mask

- 1 tablespoon of curd

- 1 tablespoon of honey

- 1 teaspoon of olive, linseed or almond (or another vegetable) oil

Knead 1 tablespoon of curd with 1 tablespoon of honey, add 1 teaspoon of olive, linseed or almond (or another vegetable) oil and stir carefully. Put this mixture on your face and neck. Wash it off at first with warm and then with cool water after 15-20 minutes.

✔ Sour cream-curd mask

- 1 tablespoon of fresh curd

- 1 tablespoon of sour cream

- 1 teaspoon of sea salt

Knead 1 tablespoon of fresh curd with 1 tablespoon of sour cream, add 1 teaspoon of sea salt and stir carefully. Put this mask on your face. Wash it off at first with warm and then with cool water after 15-20 minutes.

✔ Curd-strawberry mask

- 5-6 large strawberries
- 2 tablespoons of curd

Mash 5-6 large strawberries into gruel, add 2 tablespoons of curd and stir carefully. Put the paste on your face and leave for 10-15 minutes. Wash it off with cool water and then put a nourishing cream on your face.

✔ Curd-cucumber mask

- 2 tablespoons of fresh curd
- 1 tablespoon of milk
- 1 teaspoon of olive, sunflower or nut oil
- Cucumber
- Salt

Mix 2 tablespoons of fresh curd with 1 tablespoon of milk and 1 teaspoon of olive, sunflower or nut oil. Add a cucumber grated on a plastic grater and a pinch of salt and stir carefully. Put the mask on your face and leave for 15-20 minutes, then wash it off at first with warm and then with cool water.

✔ Yolk mask

- 1 egg yolk
- 1 teaspoon of olive or castor oil

Mix 1 egg yolk with 1 teaspoon of olive or castor oil, put this paste on your face and cover with a damp linen napkin. Leave the mask for 20 minutes and then wash it off with warm water.

✔ Yolk-carrot mask

- Carrots

- 1 egg yolk

- 1 teaspoon of sour cream

Grate carrots on a plastic grater and wring the juice out. Mix 1 egg yolk with 1 teaspoon of carrot juice and 1 teaspoon of fresh sour cream. Put this mixture on the skin of your face and leave for 15-20 minutes. Then wash the mask off at first with warm and then with cool water.

✔ Yolk-almond mask

- 1 egg yolk

- 1 tablespoon of almond oil

- Lemon essential oil

Mix the egg yolk with 1 tablespoon of almond oil and heat this mixture on a water bath. Cool it a little, add 5 drops of lemon essential oil, stir and put this warm paste on your face for 20 minutes. Wash it off at first with warm and then with cool water.

✔ Yolk-onion mask

- 1 egg yolk

- 1 tablespoon of olive or almond oil

- 1 tablespoon of onion sap

Whisk the egg yolk, mix with 1 tablespoon of olive or almond oil, add 1 tablespoon of onion sap, stir well and apply to the skin of your face for 10 minutes. Wash the mask off with warm water.

✔ Yolk-orange mask

- 1 egg yolk

- 1 tablespoon of orange juice

- 1 teaspoon of olive or any other vegetable oil

Stir the egg yolk with 1 tablespoon of orange juice and 1 teaspoon of olive or any other vegetable oil. Put this mixture on your face for 10-15 minutes, then wash it off with warm water.

✔ Egg-oatmeal mask

- 1 egg white

- 2 tablespoons of oatmeal

Whisk the egg white with 2 tablespoons of oatmeal until it is fluffy and apply to the skin of your face for 15-20 minutes. Then wash it off with warm water. This mask clears and tones skin very well.

✔ Honey mask

- Honey

Cleanse your face and apply honey heated on a water bath. Wash the mask off in 15 minutes with the help of a cotton wool ball at first with warm and then with cool water.

✔ Honey mask with green tea

- 2.5 tablespoons of honey

- 1 tablespoon of green tea

Mix 2.5 tablespoons of honey and 1 tablespoon of green tea and put the mixture on your face. Leave the mask for 20 minutes, then wash it off with warm water and rinse the face with cold water.

✔ Aloe mask

- 1 egg white

- 1 teaspoon of biostimulating aloe juice

Beat the egg white with 1 tablespoon of biostimulating aloe juice until it is fluffy and put on the skin of your face. Leave the mask for 15 minutes. It has a freshening, calming and toning effect.

✔ Oat flake mask 1

- 2 tablespoons of oat flakes

- 4-5 tablespoons of milk

- 1 teaspoon of honey

- 1 tablespoon of vegetable oil

Mix 2 tablespoons of oat flakes with 4-5 tablespoons of hot milk, add 1 teaspoon of honey and 1 tablespoon of vegetable oil. Put this paste on your face for 15-20 minutes. Wash it off with cool water.

✔ Oat flake mask 2

- 2 tablespoons of oat flakes

- 5 tablespoons of boiling water

- 1 tablespoon of olive, almond or sunflower oil

- 5 drops of lemon juice

Mix 2 tablespoons of oat flakes with 5 tablespoons of boiling water and add 1 tablespoon of olive, almond or sunflower oil and 5 drops of lemon juice. Stir the mixture carefully and apply to your skin while it is still warm. Leave the mask for 15-20 minutes on your face, then wash it off with cool water.

✔ Oat flake mask 3

- 1 tablespoon of oat flakes

- 1 tablespoon of honey

- 10 drops of lemon juice

Mix 1 tablespoon of oat flakes with 1 tablespoon of honey, add 10 drops of lemon juice and put this mixture on your face. Leave the mask for 15 minutes, then wash it off with cool water.

✔ Carrot mask 1

- 1 carrot

- 1 egg white

- 1 tablespoon of starch

Grate peeled carrot on a small plastic grater, add whipped egg white and 1 tablespoon of starch. Stir this paste carefully and put on your face. Leave the mask for 15-20 minutes, then wash it off with cool water.

✔ Carrot mask 2

- 2 small carrots

- 2 tablespoons of oatmeal

- Half a teaspoon of lemon juice

Grate two small carrots on a small plastic grater, mix with 2 tablespoons of oatmeal and add half a teaspoon of lemon juice. Put this mask on the skin of your face, leave for 20 minutes, then wash it off with cool water.

✔ Carrot mask 3

- 2 small carrots

- 1 egg yolk

- 2 tablespoons of wheat flour

Grate two small carrots on a small plastic grater, then mix with the egg yolk and 2 tablespoons of wheat flour. Put this mask on the skin of your face, leave for 20 minutes and wash it off at first with warm water, then with cool water.

✔ Sauerkraut mask 1

- Sauerkraut

- Vegetable oil

Grease your face with vegetable oil and put a layer of previously cleansed chopped sauerkraut on your skin. Leave the mask for 15-20 minutes, then wash it off with cool water.

This mask tones and freshens skin, having a rejuvenating effect.

✔ Sauerkraut mask 2

- 1 egg yolk

- 2 teaspoons of olive oil

- 2 teaspoons of sauerkraut brine

Mix the egg yolk with 2 teaspoons of olive oil and 2 teaspoons of sauerkraut brine. Put this mask on the skin of your face, leave for 15-20 minutes and wash it off at first with warm water, then with cool water. This mask tones and freshens skin, having a rejuvenating effect.

✔ Sauerkraut mask 3

- 2 tablespoons of sauerkraut

- 1 egg white

- 1 tablespoon of starch

Add 1 egg white and 1 tablespoon of starch to 2 tablespoons of sauerkraut chopped in a mincer. Stir carefully and put this mask on the face. Leave for 15-20 minutes, then wash it off with cool water. This mask tones and freshens skin, having a rejuvenating effect.

✔ Cabbage mask 4

- Fresh cabbage

Put minced cabbage gruel on your face for 20 minutes, then wash it off with room temperature water. Use for cleansing, moistening and nourishing normal skin.

✔ Potato mask

- 1 potato
- Milk or any vegetable juice

Boil the potato and mash it, adding milk or any vegetable juice. Put this mask on the skin of your face, leave for 20-25 minutes and wash it off, at first with warm water, then with cool water.

✔ Plum mask

- 2-3 ripe plums
- 1 teaspoon of fresh sour cream or vegetable oil (almond, peach, olive)
- 2 teaspoons of rye flour

Mash the pulp of 2-3 ripe plums, add 1 teaspoon of fresh sour cream or vegetable oil (almond, peach, olive) and 2 teaspoons of rye flour. Put this mask on the skin of your face, leave for 20-30 minutes and wash it off with warm water.

✔ Peach mask 1

- 1 ripe peach
- 1 teaspoon of potato starch

Mash the pulp of a ripe peach, mix with 1 teaspoon of potato starch and put it on your face. Leave for 20-30 minutes and wash it off with warm water.

✔ Peach mask 2

- 1 ripe peach

- 1 tablespoon of curd

- 1 egg yolk

Mash the pulp of a ripe peach, then add 1 tablespoon of curd and the egg yolk. Leave this mask on your face for 15 minutes and wash it off with warm water.

✔ **Peach mask 3**

- 1 peach

Slice the peach and put the slices on your face for 15-20 minutes, then rinse your face with warm water.

✔ **Apple mask**

- 1 apple

- 1 teaspoon of fresh sour cream

- 1 teaspoon of oat flour

Grate the apple on a small plastic grater, mix with 1 teaspoon of fresh sour cream and 1 teaspoon of oat flour and put this mask on the skin of your face. Leave for 20 minutes and wash it off with warm water.

✔ **Apple mask with rose petals**

- 1 apple

- 1 teaspoon of honey

- 10 fresh rose petals

- Boiled water

- 2-3 drops of lemon essential oil

Peel the apple and grate on a small plastic grater. Add 1 teaspoon of honey and 10 fresh rose petals. Add a little of boiling water and stir the mixture to a pulp consistency. Let it infuse for 20 minutes, then add 2-3 drops of lemon essential oil and put this mask on your face. Leave for 15 minutes, then wash it off with warm water. This mask tones skin, giving it a fresh and healthy appearance.

✔ Watermelon mask

- 1 teaspoon of watermelon juice

- 1 egg yolk

- 1 teaspoon of vegetable oil

Mix 1 teaspoon of watermelon juice with the egg yolk and 1 teaspoon of vegetable oil. Add rye flour until it forms a thick gruel. Put this mixture on your face for 10-15 minutes, then wash it off with cool water or chamomile tincture. The mask is recommended for normal skin inclined to dryness.

✔ Melon mask

- 2 tablespoons of melon pulp

- 1 teaspoon of honey

- 1 teaspoon of cream

Mix 2 tablespoons of melon pulp with 1 teaspoon of honey and 1 teaspoon of cream. Put this paste on your face. Leave for 15-20 minutes, then wash it off with soft warm water. This mask nourishes and tones skin.

✔ Currant mask

- 1 tablespoon of black or red currant juice

- 1 tablespoon of potato starch

Mix 1 tablespoon of black or red currant juice with 1 tablespoon of potato starch. Put this mixture on the skin of your face, leave for 15-20 minutes, then wash it off with warm water. This mask is useful for normal skin inclined to oiliness.

✔ Raspberry mask

- Raspberries

- 1 egg

Add the whipped egg to mashed raspberries and put the mixture on your face. Leave for 20 minutes, then wash it off with cool water.

✔ Banana mask 1

- 1 ripe banana

- 2 tablespoons of kefir or natural yoghurt

Mash the pulp of one ripe banana, mix with 2 tablespoons of kefir or natural yoghurt and put this mixture on the skin of your face. Leave for 10-15 minutes, then wash it off with warm water and rinse the face with cool water.

✔ Banana mask 2

- 1 ripe banana

- 1 egg white

- Half a teaspoon of peach, almond or nut oil

Mash the pulp of one ripe banana, mix with a whipped egg white, add half a teaspoon of peach, almond or nut oil and put this mixture on your face. Leave for 15 minutes, then wash it off with warm water. It tones, freshens and slightly bleaches skin.

✔ Banana mask 3

- 1 banana

- 2 tablespoons of cream

- 1 teaspoon of honey

Mash the banana to pulp, add 2 tablespoons of cream and 1 teaspoon of honey and stir carefully. Put this mixture on your face for 20 minutes, then wash it off. This mask nourishes and smoothes skin well.

✔ Pear mask

- 1 ripe pear
- 1 tablespoon of olive oil

Add 1 tablespoon of olive oil to 2 tablespoons of a ripe pear grated on a small plastic grater. Put this mask on your face for 15-20 minutes. Wash it off with warm water.

✔ Aloe and carrot mask

- 1 small carrot
- 1 tablespoon of mashed aloe
- Half a glass of concentrated tutsan extract (40 g of tutsan herb per 200 ml of water, boil for several minutes).

Peel and grate 1 small carrot on a small plastic grater, add 1 tablespoon of mashed aloe and half a glass of concentrated tutsan extract. Spread an equal layer of the resulting gruel on a piece of gauze and place on your face for 15-20 minutes, then rinse your face with warm water.

✔ Aloe mask with beet

- 1 beet
- 1 tablespoon of aloe
- 3 tablespoons of fresh milk
- 4 tablespoons of tutsan tincture (40 g of tutsan herb per 200 ml of water, infuse).

Wash the beet and boil for two hours, then cool it, peel and grate on a small grater, add 1 tablespoon of aloe. Pour 3 tablespoons of fresh milk into the gruel and add 4 tablespoons of tutsan tincture. Stir the mixture. Put it on your face for 10 minutes. Wash it off with warm water and apply cream to your face.

✔ Walnut mask

- 3-4 walnuts

- 2 tablespoons of ashberry juice

- 2 tablespoons of dried, crushed plantain grass

- 2 tablespoons of tutsan

Shell and crush 3-4 walnuts. Add 2 tablespoons of ashberry juice, 2 tablespoons of dried, crushed plantain grass and 2 tablespoons of tutsan, add water and bring to a boil. Cool and filter the resulting extract. Mix the extract with nuts and ashberry juice. Put the mask on your face. Wash it off with warm water in 20 minutes.

✔ Flower mask

- 1 tablespoon of linden flowers

- 1 tablespoon of chamomile flowers

- 200 ml of water

- 1 teaspoon of honey

- Oatmeal

Take 1 tablespoon of linden flowers and 1 tablespoon of chamomile flowers and add 200 ml of water, bring to a boil and boil on a low heat for 10 minutes. Then cool it a little and filter. Dissolve 1 teaspoon of honey in the extract and add oatmeal until it reaches the consistency of thick sour cream. Put this mixture on your face, leave for 20 minutes, then wash it off with warm water.

✔ Aloe and rose petal mask

- 1 tablespoon of aloe

- 1 tablespoon of rose petals

- 2 tablespoons of fresh chamomile flowers

- 2 tablespoons of tutsan

- 1 tablespoon of linden flowers

- Half a tablespoon of peppermint leaves

- Greasy cream

Mix and crush 1 tablespoon of aloe, 1 tablespoon of rose petals, 2 tablespoons of fresh chamomile flowers, 2 tablespoons of tutsan, 1 tablespoon of linden flowers and half a tablespoon of peppermint leaves. Put this mixture on your face, having spread cream first. Wash the mask off with warm water in 15 minutes.

✔ Tangerine mask

- 1 average tangerine

Peel the tangerine and squeeze the juice out. You can wipe the skin of your face with a cotton wool ball moistened in this juice or wet a thin layer of cotton wool or a napkin made from several layers of gauze in it and cover your face and neck with it for 15-20 minutes. After removing the mask wipe your skin at first with a damp cotton ball, and then with a dry one. You can carry out this procedure two to three times a week. A full course comprises 15-20 masks.

Creams and oils for normal facial skin

✔ Cleopatra's cream

- 40 ml of aloe juice

- 40 ml of distilled water

- 20 ml of rose water

- 10 g of honey

- 100 g of unsalted pork fat

Mix 40 ml of aloe juice, 40 ml of distilled water, 20 ml of rose water and 10 g of honey. Place this mixture on a water bath and add 100 g of unsalted pork fat to it gradually. As soon as the pork fat is rendered, remove the mixture from the water bath (be sure not to overheat it), stir well, let it cool and place into a jar. Store the cream in a refrigerator. Apply a thin layer of this cream to your face and neck once a day.

✔ Plum cream

- 1 egg yolk

- 1 teaspoon of honey

- 1 tablespoon of fresh butter

- 1 teaspoon of plum pulp

Mix the egg yolk carefully with 1 teaspoon of honey and 1 tablespoon of fresh butter. Add 1 teaspoon of plum pulp and stir. Put this cream on your face and remove the rest of it with a soft napkin in 20-30 minutes.

✔ Wild strawberry cream

- 1 egg yolk

- 2 teaspoons of fresh butter

- Half a teaspoon of honey

- 4-5 wild strawberries, pulped

Mix the egg yolk carefully with half a teaspoon of honey and 2 tablespoons of fresh butter, then add 2 teaspoons of wild strawberry pulp. Put this cream on your face and neck for 20-30 minutes, then remove the rest of it with a napkin. This cream can be stored for no longer than one hour, so you should prepare it shortly before application.

✔ Strawberry cream

- 50 ml of fresh strawberry juice

- Half a tablespoon of lanolin

- 1 tablespoon of oatmeal

Wring 50 ml of juice out of fresh strawberries. Melt half a tablespoon of lanolin on a water bath and add it to the strawberry juice. Then add 1 tablespoon of oatmeal and stir well to a homogeneous mass. Apply the cream to your face (having cleaned it first), leave for 20-30 minutes, then remove with a soft napkin.

✔ Ashberry cream

- 1 egg yolk

- 1 teaspoon of honey

- 1 tablespoon of fresh butter

- 1 tablespoon of mashed red ashberries

Mix 1 egg yolk carefully with 1 teaspoon of honey, add 1 tablespoon of fresh butter and 1 tablespoon of mashed red ashberries. Stir and put this cream on your face for 20 minutes. Remove with a soft napkin.

✔ Persimmon cream

- 1 ripe persimmon, pulped

- 1 tablespoon of butter

- 1 egg yolk

- 1 teaspoon of honey

Mix 1 tablespoon of persimmon pulp with 1 tablespoon of fresh butter, add the egg yolk and 1 teaspoon of honey and stir thoroughly. Apply the cream to your face (having cleaned it first). Remove with a soft napkin after 30 minutes.

✔ Apple cream

- 1 egg yolk

- 1 teaspoon of honey

- 1 tablespoon of butter

- 1 apple, pulped

Whisk the egg yolk with 1 teaspoon of honey and mix with about 1 tablespoon of fresh butter. Add 1 tablespoon of fresh apple pulp and stir until you get a homogeneous mass. Put a thin layer of this cream on a facial skin. Remove with a napkin after 30 minutes.

✔ Chamomile cream

- 25 g of butter

- 1 teaspoon of castor oil

- 1 teaspoon of glycerin

- 2 teaspoons of camphor spirit

- 5 teaspoons of chamomile tincture (add 1 tablespoon of chamomile flowers to 50 ml of boiling water, leave to infuse for two hours and filter)

Melt 25 g of fresh butter on a water bath and add 1 teaspoon of castor oil, 1 teaspoon of glycerin, 5 teaspoons of chamomile tincture and 2 teaspoons of camphor spirit while stirring slowly. Stir well and let it cool down. This cream is recommended for normal skin inclined to dryness.

✔ White lily oil

- 150 g of white lily blossom

- Half a liter of vegetable oil

Crush 150 g of white lily blossom and add to the vegetable oil in a glass jar. Leave to infuse for 3 weeks, shaking periodically. Then filter and store in a refrigerator. This oil makes skin smooth and silky.

Skin care recipes for oily facial skin

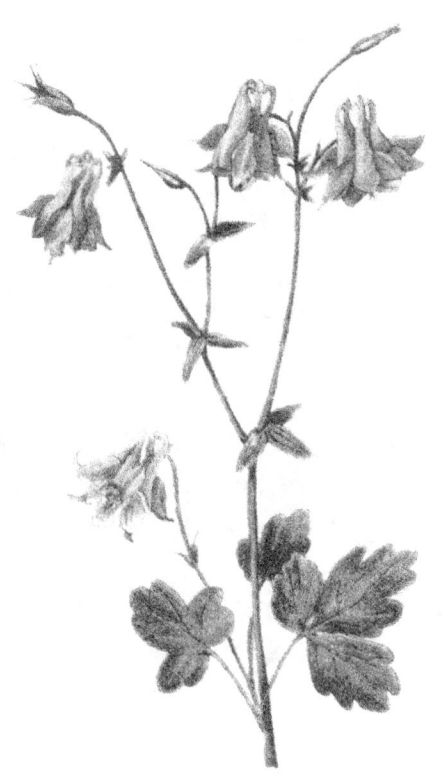

Oily facial skin

Oily skin is characterized by excessive shine due to increased greasiness and insufficient blood supply. It is inclined to the occurrence of spots and acne and sometimes looks impure. It tends to have large, clearly visible pores quite often closed by black spots. Oily skin is rather rough, and becomes especially oily and inflamed before periods. But oily skin has a great advantage compared to the other types: it is rather insensitive, meaning it remains youthful for a long time. A lot of sebum creates a protective film which does not allow moisture to evaporate and blocks penetration of harmful substances. And one more positive peculiarity: the condition of oily skin only improves over the years and becomes mixed approximately at the age of 30.

The most important action for oily skin is regular cleansing using products for normalizing the activity of sebaceous glands and increasing infection resistance. Cleanse oily skin twice a day.

Use dairy products or oat flakes to wash your face in the morning and in the evening. After washing wipe your skin with a lotion, a tea brew, calendula, sage, oak bark or coltsfoot water tincture.

Moisturizing and nourishing creams are necessary for oily skin every day. Applying bleaching and cleansing masks twice a week is recommended.

Oily facial skin cleansing

✓ **Peeling with oat flakes 1**

- 1 glass of oat flakes

- 1 teaspoon of baking soda

- Low-fat kefir or curdled milk

Add 1 teaspoon of baking soda to 1 glass of oat flakes, mix well and keep in tightly sealed glassware. Add a little low-fat kefir or curdled milk to 1 tablespoon of this mixture, stir to the consistency of gruel and rub it into the skin of your face with massaging movements. Then wash it off with warm water and rinse the face with cold water acidified with lemon juice.

✔ Peeling with oat flakes 2

- Ground oat flakes

- Green grape

Mix ground oat flakes with crushed berries of green grape to the consistency of thick gruel. Apply it to your face and rub it in with circular massaging movements. Then wash it off with warm water and rinse your face with cold water. This procedure cleanses and narrows pores, making oily skin fresh and elastic.

✔ Cleaning with salt

- Soap

- Table salt

Moisten a damp cotton wool ball with soapsuds, sprinkle with table salt and wipe your face with circular movements. Then wash it off with warm water. This procedure should be carried out two to three times a week.

✔ Cleaning with mineral water

- 200 ml of mineral water

- 1 tablespoon of grapefruit juice

Add 1 tablespoon of grapefruit juice to 200 ml of mineral water and wipe your face with it.

✔ Cleaning with dairy products

- Whey (kefir, curdled milk)

Moisten a cotton wool ball with whey (kefir or curdled milk) and apply to the oily skin of your face for the night. Do not wash the whey off at the end of the procedure, but remove it with a well-wrung cotton ball.

✔ Cleaning with lemon

- Lemon

You can wipe your oily skin with a slice of lemon in the morning and in the evening. Fifteen to twenty minutes after cleaning, apply a light cream to your face. Oily porous skin is cleaned well with pure lemon juice. If your skin is inclined to irritation, you can dilute it with water.

✔ Cleaning with mint ice

- 1 tablespoon of peppermint leaves

- 200 ml of water

- 1 teaspoon of lemon juice

Add 1 tablespoon of peppermint leaves to 200 ml of water, heat on a water bath for 15 minutes, let it infuse for 45 minutes and filter. Add 1 teaspoon of lemon juice to this mint tincture and freeze it in ice moulds. Wipe oily skin with a cube of mint ice with slight circular movements in the morning, and then apply a thin layer of cream. This procedure moistens and tones skin.

✔ Cleaning with pea paste

- 1 tablespoon of pea flour

- 1 teaspoon of oatmeal

- Pinch of ground cinnamon

- Rose water

Mix 1 tablespoon of pea flour with 1 teaspoon of oatmeal and a pinch of ground cinnamon. Dilute the mixture with rose water to the consistency of paste and apply to your face. Wash it off with warm water after 10 minutes. This mixture clears skin perfectly.

Tinctures for oily facial skin cleansing

✔ Calendula tincture

- 40 g of calendula flowers

- 200 ml of vodka

Add 40 g of calendula blossom to 200 ml of vodka, leave to infuse for two weeks in a dark place and then filter the tincture and wipe the skin of your face with it.

Warning:

Use calendula carefully if you suffer from allergies.

✔ Tutsan tincture

- 40 g of tutsan grass

- 200 ml of vodka

Add 40 g of crushed tutsan grass to 200 ml of vodka, leave to infuse in a dark place for two weeks, then filter and use this tincture for cleaning of your skin.

Warning:

Tutsan makes skin more sensitive to ultraviolet rays. Use tutsan tinctures with care during the summer.

✔ Field horsetail tincture

- 20 g of crushed field horsetail grass

- 200 ml of vodka

Add 20 g of crushed field horsetail grass to 200 ml of vodka, leave to infuse in a dark place for two weeks, then filter and use for cleaning the skin of your face.

✔ Arnica tincture

- 20 g of mountain arnica
- 200 ml of vodka

Add 20 g of mountain arnica to 200 ml of vodka, leave to infuse in a dark place for 7-10 days, filter and wipe the skin of your face.

✔ Chamomile tincture

- 20 g of chamomile flowers
- 200 ml of vodka

Add 20 g of chamomile flowers to 200 ml of vodka, leave to infuse in a dark place for 7-10 days and filter. Wipe oily skin with this tincture.

✔ Cinquefoil tincture

- 2 tablespoons of crushed cinquefoil rhizome
- 200 ml of vodka

Add 2 tablespoons of crushed cinquefoil rhizome to 200 ml of vodka, leave to infuse for two weeks in a dark place, filter and use for skin cleaning.

✔ Sophora tincture

- Crushed sophora japonica fruits
- Vodka

Add crushed sophora japonica fruits to the vodka at a 1:5 proportion, leave to infuse, shaking periodically, in a dark place for 10 days and filter. Use for cleaning the skin of your face.

✔ Herbal tincture

- Peppermint leaves
- Nettle leaves
- Sage leaves
- Bur-marigold herb
- Yarrow herb
- Calendula blossom
- 200ml of vodka
- Water

Mix equal parts of peppermint leaves, nettle leaves, sage leaves, bur marigold herb, yarrow herb and calendula blossom. Add 40 g of the mixture to 200ml of vodka and leave to infuse in a dark place for two weeks. Filter it and dilute with water (1:5) before application.

✔ Rose tincture

- 20 g of dried rose petals
- 200 ml of vodka

Add 20 g of dried rose petals to 200 ml of vodka (or fill a bottle with fresh petals and then fill it with vodka to the brim) and leave to infuse in a dark place for two weeks, stirring every day. Then filter the mixture and keep in a tightly sealed vessel. Wipe your porous skin with this tincture. It possesses astringent and antiseptic action, preventing the occurrence of wrinkles.

✔ Wild strawberry tincture

- Wild strawberries

- 200 ml of vodka

- Water

Mash the wild strawberries, then add half a glass of berry pulp to 200 ml of vodka. Leave to infuse for one month. Then filter, dilute with water at a 1:1 ratio and use to wipe the oily skin of your face.

✔ **Quince tincture**

- 1 quince

- 200 ml of vodka

Chop 1 quince, add it to 200 ml of vodka and let it infuse for 7-10 days. Then filter the tincture and use it for cleaning the oily skin of your face.

Herbal tinctures and extracts for oily facial skin

✔ **Bluebottle tincture**

- 2 tablespoons of bluebottle marginal flowers

- 200 ml of water

Add 2 tablespoons of bluebottle marginal flowers to 200 ml of water, heat on a water bath for 15 minutes, let it infuse for 45 minutes and filter. This infusion is useful for oily skin with large pores.

✔ **Plantain extract**

- 1-2 tablespoons of plantain leaves

- 200 ml of water

Add 1-2 tablespoons of plantain leaves to 200 ml of water, heat on a water bath for 30 minutes, let it cool for 10 minutes and filter. Use this extract for cleaning the oily skin of your face.

✔ Oak bark extract

- 10-20 g of crushed oak bark

- Water

Use a 5-10 % oak bark extract for wiping and washing oily porous skin inclined to acne. Put 10-20 g of crushed bark into an enameled pot, fill it with a glass of water and close with a cover. Boil the mixture on a low heat or a water bath for 30 minutes, filter it and add boiled water to the initial volume. This extract promotes reduction of sebaceous excretions, narrows pores and makes your skin resilient and elastic.

✔ Bur-marigold herb tincture

- 2-3 tablespoons of crushed bur-marigold herb

- Half a liter of water

Add 2-3 tablespoons of crushed bur-marigold herb to half a liter of water, heat on a water bath for 15 minutes, let it infuse for 45 minutes, filter and then wipe skin inclined to inflammations with this tincture.

✔ Nettle tincture

- 2 tablespoons of crushed nettle leaves

- 200 ml of boiling water

Add 2 tablespoons of crushed nettle leaves to 200 ml of boiling water, leave to infuse in a closed vessel for 30 minutes and filter. Wipe the oily skin of your face with this tincture. It can also be used for compresses.

✔ Arnica and sage tincture

- 1 tablespoon of mountain arnica

- 1 tablespoon of sage leaves

- 200 ml of water

Add 1 tablespoon of mountain arnica and 1 tablespoon of sage leaves to 200 ml of water, heat on a water bath for 15 minutes, let it infuse for 45 minutes at room temperature, filter and wipe your oily skin with this infusion.

✔ **Hop tincture**

- 1 tablespoon of crushed hops
- 200 ml of boiling water

Add 1 tablespoon of crushed hops to 200 ml of boiling water, leave to infuse for two hours in a closed pan at room temperature and filter. Wipe your face with this infusion. It can also be used for compresses.

✔ **Peppermint and plantain tincture**

- Half a glass of fresh peppermint leaves
- Half a glass of dried or fresh plantain leaves
- 400 ml of boiling water

Add half a glass of fresh crushed peppermint leaves and the same amount of crushed dried or fresh plantain leaves to 400 ml of boiling water and put in warm place for two to three hours.

The tincture is recommended for wiping oily skin.

Lotions, toilet water and milk for oily facial skin

✔ **Aloe lotion**

- 200 ml of aloe juice
- 50 ml of vodka

Mix 200 ml of aloe juice with about 50 ml of vodka and use for facial cleansing. Keep this lotion in a cool, dark place in a tightly sealed vessel.

✔ Lemon lotion 1

- 1 lemon juice
- 100 ml of vodka

Mix the lemon juice with the vodka and use for cleansing oily skin.

✔ Lemon lotion 2

- 1 egg white
- Lemon juice (2 lemons)
- 50 ml of cologne
- 1 teaspoon of glycerin
- A pinch of salt

Whip the egg white, adding the lemon juice. Pour the mixture into a bottle and add the cologne, glycerin and salt. Wipe the skin of your face with this lotion for the night. It narrows pores well, and if necessary, you may rinse your face with warm baking soda water to soften skin (half a teaspoon of baking soda per half a liter of water). Keep this lotion in a refrigerator, and shake before use.

✔ Lemon-cranberry lotion

- 1 lemon
- 100 ml of vodka
- 100 ml of cranberry juice
- 50 ml of distilled water
- Half a tablespoon of glycerin

Grate half a lemon with peel on a plastic grater, add 100 ml of vodka and leave to infuse in a dark place for a week. Then filter, add 100 ml of cranberry juice and 50 ml of distilled water, half a tablespoon of glycerin and mix carefully. Wipe the skin of your face with this lotion for the night. A full course comprises two to three weeks. Keep this lotion in a refrigerator.

✔ **Lemon lotion with viburnum juice**

- Lemon juice (1 lemon)

- 2 tablespoons of viburnum juice

- 1 egg white

- 1 teaspoon of glycerin

- 100 ml of vodka

Mix the lemon juice with 2 tablespoons of viburnum juice and egg white. Add 1 teaspoon of glycerin and 100 ml of vodka and wipe your skin with the lotion.

✔ **Cucumber lotion 1**

- 1 small fresh cucumber

- Vodka

Grate the cucumber on a plastic grater and pour with the same volume of vodka. Leave to infuse for two weeks in a closed vessel, filter and use for cleaning oily skin. This lotion possesses bleaching and astringent effects.

✔ **Cucumber lotion 2**

- 50 g of fresh cucumber peel

- 250 ml of water

Crush 50 g of fresh cucumber peel, add 250 ml of warm water and let it infuse for six hours. Then filter it and use to wipe your skin several times a day.

✔ **Watermelon lotion**

- Watermelon pulp

- Half a tablespoon of honey

- Half a teaspoon of salt

- 100 ml of vodka

Mash the watermelon pulp and wring 250 ml of juice out. Add the honey and salt and stir well. When the salt dissolves, filter the mixture and add 100 ml of vodka. This lotion can be stored in a refrigerator for six months. It clears and moistens skin well.

✔ Orange lotion

- 1 orange

- 100 ml of vodka

- 1 tablespoon of rose petal tincture or rose water

- 1 teaspoon of glycerin

Grate 1 orange with peel on a plastic grater and add 100 ml of vodka. Infuse inside dark glassware in a warm place for a week, then filter this mixture and add 1 tablespoon of rose petal tincture or rose water and 1 teaspoon of glycerin. Store this lotion in a refrigerator.

✔ Grapefruit lotion

- 200 ml of grapefruit juice

- 1 tablespoon of lemon juice

- 1 tablespoon of vodka

- 2 tablespoons of distilled water

Mix 200 ml of grapefruit juice with 1 tablespoon of lemon juice and 1 tablespoon of vodka. Add 2 tablespoons of distilled water, pour the mixture into a glassware container and close it tightly. Shake before use.

✔ Strawberry lotion

- 100 ml of strawberry juice

- 100 ml of vodka

Mix 100 ml of strawberry juice with about 100 ml of vodka and use for skin cleansing. If your skin is too sensitive, it's a good idea to dilute the lotion with some water.

✓ **Quince lotion**

- 1 quince

- 200 ml of vodka

Chop the quince into small slices, add 200 ml of vodka and leave to infuse in a dark place for 7-10 days. Then filter and use for cleaning oily skin with large pores.

✓ **Elder flowers lotion**

- 1 tablespoon of dried common elder flowers

- 200 ml of water

- 2 tablespoons of onion juice

- 6 tablespoons of cucumber juice

- 4 tablespoons of cologne

Add 1 tablespoon of dried common elder blossom to 200 ml of water, heat on a water bath for 15 minutes, let it infuse for 45 minutes and filter. Add two tablespoons of onion juice, six tablespoons of cucumber juice and four tablespoons of cologne into the tincture and wipe your oily skin with it (suitable for normal skin as well).

✓ **Rose lotion**

- 150 ml of rose water

- 50 ml of young hazel extract (1 tablespoon of crushed young branches, 200 ml of water)

Mix 150 ml of rose water with about 50 ml of young hazel extract (to prepare the extract add 1 tablespoon of crushed young branches to 200 ml of water, heat on a water bath in a closed vessel for 30 minutes, filter and let it cool). Wipe your face with the lotion. If your skin is very oily, use rose water and hazel extract in equal parts. This lotion possesses cleansing and astringent properties, and freshens and tones skin.

✔ Coltsfoot lotion

- 2 tablespoons of dried coltsfoot leaves
- 250 ml of water
- Vodka

Add 2 tablespoons of dried coltsfoot leaves to 250 ml of water, heat in a sealed vessel on a water bath for 15 minutes, let it infuse for 45 minutes and filter. Add vodka (4:1) and wipe oily porous skin with the lotion.

✔ Bluebottle flowers lotion

- 1 tablespoon of bluebottle marginal flowers
- 200 ml of water
- 1 teaspoon of vodka

Add 1 tablespoon of bluebottle marginal flowers to 200 ml of water, heat on a water bath for 15 minutes, let it infuse for 45 minutes and filter. Mix this infusion with one teaspoon of vodka and wipe oily skin with large pores with this lotion two to three times a day.

✔ Linden lotion with aromatic oils

- 1 tablespoon of linden bark
- 200 ml of water
- Pinch of crushed willow bark
- 4 tablespoons of rose water
- 1 tablespoon of honey

- 5 drops of lavender oil

- 2-3 drops of carnation oil

Add 1 tablespoon of linden bark to 200 ml of water, heat on a water bath for 15 minutes, let it infuse for 30 minutes and filter. Mix 120 ml of the linden infusion and a pinch of crushed willow bark in a piece of glassware and add 4 tablespoons of rose water, 1 tablespoon of honey, 5 drops of lavender oil, 2-3 drops of carnation oil. Close the vessel tightly and leave to infuse for 2 weeks, stirring every day. This lotion possesses effective astringent action.

✔ Nettle lotion 1

- 1 glass of fresh nettle leaves

- 200 ml of vodka

- 30 ml of distilled water

Add 1 glass of crushed fresh nettle leaves to 200 ml of vodka and leave to infuse in tightly sealed glassware in a dark place for 10 days. Then filter it, add 30 ml of distilled water and wipe your skin with the lotion.

✔ Nettle lotion 2

- 100 ml of vodka

- 1 tablespoon of fresh nettle juice

Add 100 ml of vodka to 1 tablespoon of fresh nettle juice and wipe oily skin in the morning and in the evening.

✔ Tutsan lotion

- 1 tablespoon of tutsan tincture (40 g of tutsan, 200 ml of vodka)

- Half a teaspoon of honey

- 2 teaspoons of fresh apple juice

- 5 g of yeast

- Water

Mix 1 tablespoon of tutsan tincture (add 40 g of crushed tutsan herb to 200 ml of vodka, leave to infuse in a dark place for 2 weeks, then filter) with half a teaspoon of honey and 2 teaspoons of fresh apple juice. Add 5 g of yeast, broken in a small amount of warm water. Wipe oily skin with this lotion. Rinse your face with cool water after 10 minutes.

✔ Face-washing composition with tea mushroom tincture

- Mineral water

- Tea mushroom tincture

Mix mineral water with tea mushroom tincture (1:1) and use for cleansing your face in the morning and in the evening.

✔ Lemon water

- 1 lemon

- Water

Chop the lemon, add water, let it infuse in a closed vessel for two to three hours and filter. Wipe your face with the lemon water for three to four days, then have a two week break (using other products during the time).

✔ Orange water

- 1 orange peel, chopped

- 250 ml of water

Add chopped peel to 250 ml of water and let it infuse for one day. Then filter it and use to wipe your face in the morning and in the evening. Orange water freshens and rejuvenates skin well along with narrowing pores.

✔ **Lemon milk**

- 1 slice of lemon

- Milk

Add a slice of lemon to warm milk and leave it in a closed ceramic vessel for three hours. Then put this lemon milk on your previously cleansed skin with a cotton wool ball. This ancient English recipe softens skin perfectly.

✔ **Parsley with white wine**

- 1 tablespoon of dried parsley roots and leaves

- 1 glass of boiling water

- Half a glass of white wine

Add 1 tablespoon of dried parsley roots and leaves to a glass of boiling water, boil on a water bath for 20-30 minutes, leave to infuse for an hour, filter it and add half a glass of white wine. You can use fresh parsley instead of dried as well.

Compresses for oily facial skin

Warm, hot and contrasted compresses are recommended for oily skin. Apply them – having previously cleaned your face – before massage or the application of a mask. It is recommended that you apply compresses two to three times a week. One course includes 15-20 procedures. Warm and hot compresses aren't recommended in the case of increased arterial pressure and blood vessels showing through the skin.

✔ **Compress with green tea**

- 100 ml of strong green tea

- Lemon juice

If you have oily porous skin, make 100 ml of strong green tea, add several drops of lemon juice, moisten a gauze napkin in it and put a warm compress on your face for 10-15 minutes, changing it as soon as it gets cold.

✔ Compress with chamomile tincture

- 4 tablespoons of chamomile flowers
- 200 ml of hot water

Add 4 tablespoons of chamomile flowers to 200 ml of hot water, heat on a water bath for 15 minutes, let it infuse at room temperature for 45 minutes and filter. Moisten a napkin in the warm tincture, wring it out slightly and apply to your face. Leave for five minutes. Repeat this procedure several times.

✔ Compress with peppermint tincture

- 1 tablespoon of crushed peppermint leaves
- 200 ml of boiling water

Add 1 tablespoon of crushed peppermint leaves to 200 ml of boiling water, let it infuse in a closed vessel for 20 minutes and filter. Moisten a napkin in the warm tincture and apply to your face. Leave for 15-20 minutes. This compress freshens oily skin well.

✔ Compress with tutsan decoction

- 1.5 tablespoons of tutsan herb
- 200 ml of water

Add 1.5 tablespoons of tutsan herb to 200 ml of water, heat on a water bath for 30 minutes and filter. Moisten a napkin in the warm tincture, apply to your face and leave for 15 minutes, changing it as soon as it gets cold.

✓ **Compress with cinquefoil extract**

- 1 tablespoon of crushed cinquefoil rhizomes

- 200 ml of water

Add 1 tablespoon of crushed cinquefoil rhizomes to 200 ml of water, heat on a water bath for 30 minutes, filter and let it cool. Moisten a gauze napkin in the warm tincture, apply to your face and leave for 15 minutes. This compress is useful for oily skin with enlarged pores.

✓ **Compress with yarrow tincture**

- 2 tablespoons of yarrow herb

- 400 ml of water

Add 2 tablespoons of yarrow herb to 400 ml of water, heat on a water bath for 15 minutes, let it infuse for 45 minutes and filter. Cool half of it in a refrigerator, warm the other half and make contrast compresses, moistening napkins in turns with warm and cold tinctures. The last compress should be cold. Yarrow tincture clears pores well. Another option is applying only a warm compress several times.

✓ **Compress with field horsetail extract**

- 1-2 tablespoons of field horsetail herb

- 200 ml of water

Add 1-2 tablespoons of field horsetail herb to 200 ml of water, heat on a water bath for 30 minutes, let it cool for 10 minutes and filter. Moisten a napkin in the warm extract and apply the compress to your face. Leave it for five minutes. Repeat this procedure several times. You can make the same compresses with a sage leave tincture.

✓ **Compress with herbal tincture**

- Dandelion leaves

- Plantain leaves

- Sage leaves

- Bur-marigold herb

- Chamomile flowers

- 200 ml of water

Mix the leaves of dandelion, plantain, sage, bur-marigold herb and chamomile flowers in equal parts. Add 1 tablespoon of this mixture to 200 ml of water, heat on a water bath for 15 minutes, infuse for 45 minutes and filter. Warm this tincture, moisten a napkin in it and apply to your face. Leave until it becomes cold. Repeat this procedure several times.

✓ **Compress with sweetflag extract for oily skin**

- 2 tablespoons of crushed sweetflag rhizome

- 1 liter of water

Add 2 tablespoons of crushed sweetflag rhizome to 1 liter of cold water in an enameled pan, cover and bring to a boil on a low heat. Filter and use the moderately hot extract for applying compresses to your face and neck. To do so take a terry towel, fold it in 2-3 layers, moisten with the extract, wring it out and put it quickly on your face so that the middle of the compress falls on your chin and its sides cover your cheeks. Leave for 10-15 minutes. It is a good idea to apply such a compress before cosmetic procedures (massage, masks). Clean your skin before applying a compress. A hot compress widens pores, increases blood supply to the surface of skin, warms it and promotes removal of dust and dead cells. Skin becomes soft and gentle. However, it isn't recommended in the case of enlarged skin vessels, pustular lesions and inflammations.

Cleansing masks for oily facial skin

✓ **Mask with therapeutic mud**

- Thyme herb

- Rosemary leaves

- 200 ml of water

- 3 tablespoons of therapeutic mud

Add 1 tablespoon of thyme herb or rosemary leaves to 200 ml of water, heat on a water bath for 15 minutes, let it infuse for 45 minutes and filter. Mix 3 tablespoons of therapeutic mud with 1 teaspoon of tincture to the consistency of a thick paste. Put a thin layer of this paste on your skin (not covering the area around the eyes and lips) and leave the mask for 20 minutes. Soften the dried mask with a wet napkin, wash it off with warm water and apply a moisturizer to your face.

✔ White clay mask

- 10 g of white clay

- 1 teaspoon of rice flour

- 2 tablespoons of fresh milk

Mix 10 g of white clay and 1 teaspoon of rice flour with 2 tablespoons of fresh milk. Apply this mixture to your face and leave the mask for 15-20 minutes, then wash it off with warm water. Clay masks have clearing and drying properties. They should be applied once a week.

✔ Oat flakes mask

- 2 tablespoons of ground oat flakes

- Low-fat kefir or mineral water

- Half a teaspoon of baking soda

Stir 2 tablespoons of ground oat flakes with low-fat kefir or mineral water to the consistency of gruel, add half a teaspoon of baking soda and apply this mixture to your face with massaging movements. In 20 minutes wash this mask off at first with warm, then with lightly salted or acidified cold water. This mask clears skin well, making it elastic and smooth.

✓ Egg-oatmeal mask

- 1 egg white
- 2 tablespoons of oatmeal

Mix one egg white with 2 tablespoons of oatmeal or cornflour, whip into a froth and apply to your face. After it becomes dry, remove the mask with a dry linen napkin and rinse the face with cool water.

✓ Egg-sugar mask

- 1 egg white
- 1 tablespoon of sugar

Whisk one egg white with 1 tablespoon of sugar into a white froth. Put part of this mixture on your skin and leave until it becomes dry. Moisten your palms with the rest of mixture and massage your skin. Continue this procedure until the palms begin sticking to the face. Then wash the mask off with cool water and apply moisture cream. This mask clears pores well. In the case of highly impure skin, you can apply this mask daily.

✓ Almond mask

- 1 tablespoon of almond bran
- 1 tablespoon of whey

Mix 1 tablespoon of almond bran with 1 tablespoon of whey and put this mixture on your face, massaging it slightly. Leave the mask for 15-20 minutes, then wash it off with cool water. The mask has a clearing and exfoliating effect.

✓ Wheat-honey mask

- 1 tablespoon of wheat sprouts

- 1 tablespoon of honey

- Half a teaspoon of rose water

- Half a teaspoon of almond oil

Mix 1 tablespoon of wheat germinants with 1 tablespoon of honey, add half a teaspoon of rose water and almond oil. Leave this mask for 10-15 minutes, then remove it with a warm wet napkin. It provides good cleansing, moistening and refreshing skin.

✔ **Rye flour and chamomile mask**

- 2 tablespoons of chamomile flowers

- Boiling water

- 1 teaspoon of lemon juice

- 2 teaspoons of rye flour

Crush 2 tablespoons of chamomile flowers and pour boiling water over. Add 1 teaspoon of lemon juice and 2 teaspoons of rye flour until a thick gruel has formed. Apply a warm mask to your face, leave for 20 minutes, then wash it off with cool water.

✔ **Rye flour mask with bluebottle decoction**

- 1 tablespoon of bluebottle marginal flowers

- 50 ml of water

- 10 drops of lemon juice

- Rye flour

Add 1 tablespoon of bluebottle marginal flowers to 50 ml of water, cover and boil for 5 minutes on a low heat, let it cool down and filter. Add 10 drops of lemon juice and rye flour, stirring to the consistency of a thick gruel and apply the mask to your face. Leave it for 20 minutes, then wash it off with cool water.

✓ Pea mask

- 2 tablespoons of pea flour

- 2 tablespoons of curdled milk or whey

Mix 2 tablespoons of pea flour with 2 tablespoons of curdled milk or whey. Apply the mask to your face and remove it with a dry cotton ball once it dries. Then rinse the face, first with warm and then with cool water.

✓ Tomato mask 1

- Fresh tomatoes

- 2 tablespoons of oat flour

Rub the tomatoes through a sieve and add the oat flour to 2 tablespoons of juice with pulp. Apply this mixture to your face. Leave it for 10-15 minutes, wash it off with warm water and then rinse it with cold water. This mask is recommended for oily skin with enlarged pores.

✓ Tomato mask 2

- 1 ripe tomato

Mash the pulp of a ripe tomato well and apply to the skin of your face. Leave it for 10 minutes, then wash it off with cool water. This mask is recommended for oily skin with enlarged pores.

✓ Tomato mask 3

- 2 tablespoons of fresh tomato juice

- 1-2 tablespoons of rye flour or corn starch

Mix 2 tablespoons of fresh tomato juice with 1-2 tablespoons of rye flour or corn starch. Leave the mask on your face for 10-15 minutes and wash it off with cool water. This mask is recommended for oily skin with enlarged pores.

✓ **Marrow squash mask**

- Marrow squash

- 1 tablespoon of steamed oat flakes

Mix 2 tablespoons of a marrow squash grated on a small plastic grater with 1 tablespoon of steamed oat flakes (with boiling water). Leave the mask for 20 minutes, wash it off with warm water, then rinse your face with cold water. This mask clears impure oily skin well.

✓ **Cucumber mask with clay**

- Half a small cucumber

- Blue clay

Grate a half of a small cucumber on a plastic grater and mix with blue clay to the consistency of gruel. Put an even layer of this mask on your face (excluding the area around the eyes and lips) and leave for 20 minutes. Wash it off with warm water and apply moisture cream to your face.

✓ **Avocado mask**

- Half an avocado

- 2 tablespoons of oat flakes

Peel a half of an avocado, mash the pulp and mix it with 2 tablespoons of oat flakes. Put this paste on your face and leave for 15-20 minutes. Then wash it off with warm water and rinse your face with cold water.

✓ **Bergenia tincture mask**

- 50 g of crushed bergenia roots

- Half a liter of vodka

- Non-greasy nourishing cream

Add 50 g of crushed bergenia roots to half a liter of vodka, leave to infuse for 30 days in a dark place, then filter. Moisten a gauze or linen napkin in this tincture and put it on your face for 15 minutes. Then apply a thin layer of non-greasy nourishing cream. Bergenia tincture cures inflammations and narrows pores. This procedure is carried out twice a week.

✔ Herbal infusion mask

- Chamomile flowers

- Linden flowers

- Elder flowers

- Half a teaspoon of honey

- Oatmeal

- Glass of boiling water

This mask is prepared with an infusion of chamomile flowers, linden flowers and elder flowers taken in equal parts, honey and oatmeal. It clears skin, narrows pores and improves blood circulation. Take 1 tablespoon of the herbal mixture, add a glass of boiling water, boil thoroughly for 10 minutes then filter. Add half a teaspoon of honey and oatmeal to the warm infusion and mix to the consistency of gruel. Put a thick layer of this mask on your face. Wash it off with warm water, then rinse the face with cool water.

✔ Carrot mask

- 1 carrot

- Starch

Mix a carrot grated on a small grater (or carrot juice) with starch to the consistency of gruel. Apply it to your face and leave for 15 minutes, then wash it off.

Moisturizing masks for oily facial skin

✔ **Dairy mask**

- 2 tablespoons of low-fat kefir

- 2 tablespoons of oatmeal

- Dandelion or plantain leaves

Mix 2 tablespoons of low-fat kefir with 2 tablespoons of oatmeal and add a small amount of crushed dandelion or plantain leaves. Leave the mask for 20 minutes, and then wash it off with warm and then with cold water. This mask moistens and softens oily skin.

✔ **Apricot mask**

- 2 tablespoons of fresh apricot pulp

- 1 tablespoon of curdled milk

Mix 2 tablespoons of fresh apricot pulp with 1 tablespoon of curdled milk. Apply the mask for 15-20 minutes, then wash it off with cool water.

✔ **Avocado mask**

- Half an avocado

- 1 egg white

- 1 teaspoon of lemon juice

Mix the avocado pulp with the egg white whipped into a froth and 1 teaspoon of lemon juice. Apply the mask for 20 minutes and then wash it off with cool water.

✔ **Honey-egg mask**

- 2 egg whites

- 30 g of honey

- Half a teaspoon of almond or peach oil

- 2 tablespoons of ground oat flakes

Mix the egg whites with the honey and oil into a homogeneous paste, then add the oat flakes. Wash the mask off, at first with warm and then with cool water. This mask moistens, nourishes and clears skin.

✔ Strawberry mask

- Lemon leaves

- Oat flakes

- 3 tablespoons of wheat sprouts

- Fresh strawberries

Boil the lemon leaves. Mix the extract with a cup of oat flakes and 3 tablespoons of wheat sprouts. Add strawberries pulp to this mixture. Apply the mask to your face and leave for one hour. Wash it off with warm water.

✔ Berry mask

- 2-3 raspberries

- 2-3 strawberries

- 1 apricot

- 1 teaspoon of grated fresh cabbage

- 1 teaspoon of cream

Mash 2-3 raspberries, 2-3 strawberries and 1 apricot, add 1 teaspoon of a grated fresh cabbage and 1 teaspoon of cream. Apply the mask to your face and leave for 15 minutes. Wash it off with cool water, then with warm and then with cool water again.

✔ Apricot with kefir

- 1 apricot

- Kefir

Mix the apricot pulp with the kefir at a 1:1 ratio and apply to your face for 20 minutes.

Astringent masks for oily facial skin

✓ Yeast mask 1

- 20 g of yeast

- Orange juice

- Mineral water

Break 20 g of yeast in a mix of orange juice and mineral water (at a 1:1 ratio) to the consistency of a thick cream. Apply the mask to your face and leave for 20 minutes. Wash it off, at first with warm and then with cold water. This mask eliminates oily shine and narrows pores.

✓ Yeast mask 2

- 20 g of yeast

- Milk

Break 20 g of yeast in warm milk to the consistency of cream and apply to the skin of your face. Leave the mask for 20 minutes. Wash it off, at first with warm and then with cold water. The mask narrows pores, softens and tones skin.

✓ Yeast mask 3

- 20 g of yeast

- 1 teaspoon of cranberry juice

- 1 teaspoon of cowberry juice

- Milk

Mix 20 g of yeast with 1 teaspoon of cranberry juice and 1 teaspoon of cowberry juice. Stir to the consistency of cream, add some milk, and apply the mask to your face. Leave for 15 minutes. Wash it off, at first with warm and then with cold water.

✔ **Egg mask**

- 1 egg

Whip the egg carefully, spread the froth on your face and leave it on your skin for 20 minutes, then wash it off with warm water.

✔ **Egg mask with aloe juice**

- 1 egg white

- 1 teaspoon of biostimulating aloe juice

Whip 1 egg white into froth, adding 1 teaspoon of biostimulating aloe juice and apply it to the skin of your face. Leave the mask for 15 minutes, then wash it off with warm water. It has an astringent and stimulating effect.

✔ **Egg mask with chamomile tincture**

- 1 egg white

- 1 teaspoon of lemon juice

- 100 ml of chamomile tincture (1 tablespoon of chamomile flowers, 100 ml of boiling water)

Whip the egg white, add 1 teaspoon of lemon juice and 100 ml of chamomile tincture (to prepare this tincture take 1 tablespoon of chamomile flowers and add it to 100 ml of boiling water, leave to infuse in a closed vessel for 1 hour), stir well and put this mixture on your face. Wash it off with cold water after 20 minutes.

✓ Egg mask with cranberry juice 1

- 1 egg white
- 1 tablespoon of cranberry juice
- Tea

Whip the egg white into froth, adding 1 tablespoon of cranberry juice little-by-little. Put the mask on your face in 2-3 layers (every following layer should be applied when the previous one has dried). Leave it for 20 minutes and remove with a cotton wool ball moistened in tea. This mask is recommended for oily skin with enlarged pores.

✓ Egg mask with cranberry juice 2

- 1 egg white
- 1 teaspoon of cranberry juice
- 1 teaspoon of corn starch

Whip the egg white into froth with 1 teaspoon of cranberry juice and 1 teaspoon of corn starch. Put this paste on the skin of your face and leave for 20 minutes. Then wash it off with cool water.

✓ Egg-lemon mask 1

- 1 egg white
- Lemon rind

Whip the egg white and add grated lemon rind. Put this mixture on your face and leave for 20 minutes, then wash it off with cool water. This mask eliminates oily shine and narrows pores well.

✓ Egg-lemon mask 2

- 1 egg white
- Half a teaspoon of lemon juice

Whip the egg white into froth, adding half a teaspoon of lemon juice. Put this mixture on your face and leave for 15-20 minutes, then wash it off with cold water and apply some moisturizing cream. This mask eliminates oily shine and narrows pores well.

✓ Almond mask with herbs

- Almond

- Herbal infusion (chamomile and linden flowers, melissa leaves, sage herb)

- 1 teaspoon of honey

Add 2 tablespoons of crushed almonds to the hot herbal tincture and stir to the consistency of gruel. Add 1 teaspoon of honey and mix carefully once again. Apply the warm mask to your face and leave for 20-30 minutes. Wash it off with warm, then cold water. This mask is useful for oily porous skin.

✓ Cucumber mask 1

- Fresh cucumber

- Tutsan, horsetail extract or calendula tincture

Place thin slices of fresh cucumber on your face and cover with a gauze napkin. Remove the mask in 15-20 minutes and leave cucumber juice on the face for 2-3 minutes. Then wash it off with warm water and make a cool compress with tutsan or horsetail extract, or calendula tincture. This mask is useful for oily porous skin, having a cleansing and astringent effect; it also slightly bleaches skin.

✓ Cucumber mask 2

- Fresh cucumber

- 1 egg white

Grate a fresh cucumber on a small plastic grater, mix with a well-whipped egg white and apply to the skin of your face.

Leave the mask for 15-20 minutes, then wash it off with cool water. This mask narrows pores well.

✔ Currant mask

- Red and white currants

- 1 tablespoon of corn starch

Mash several red and white currants well, mix with 1 tablespoon of corn starch and put this mixture on your face. Leave the mask for 15-20 minutes. Wash it off with warm and then with cold water.

✔ Apple mask 1

- 1 apple

- 1 tablespoon of milk

- 1 egg white

Peel an apple and grate on a small plastic grater. Add 1 tablespoon of milk and a whipped egg white. Stir carefully and put this mixture on the skin of your face. Leave the mask for 10-15 minutes. Wash it off with warm water.

✔ Apple mask 2

- 1 apple

- 1 tablespoon of starch

Peel an apple and grate it on a small plastic grater. Mix 2 tablespoons of apple pulp with 1 tablespoon of starch and apply the mixture to the skin of your face. Leave the mask for 15 minutes, then wash it off with cool water.

✔ Apple mask 3

- 1 apple

- 1 teaspoon of lemon juice

- 1 egg white

Grate the apple on a small grater and add 1 teaspoon of lemon juice and 1 egg white whipped into froth. Stir carefully and apply this mixture to the skin of your face. Leave the mask for 10 minutes, then wash it off with cool water.

✔ Quince mask 1

- Quince

- 1 egg white

Quince freshens skin and possesses fine astringent action. Mix 2 tablespoons of quince, peeled and grated on a small plastic grater, with 1 egg white whipped into froth. Apply the mask for 15-20 minutes, then rinse your face with warm water.

✔ Quince mask 2

- Quince

- 1 tablespoon of kefir

- 1 teaspoon of honey

Mix 2 tablespoons of quince, grated on a small grater, with 1 tablespoon of kefir and 1 teaspoon of honey. Apply this mixture to the skin of your face for 20 minutes. Then wash it off with warm water and rinse with cold water.

✔ Horse sorrel mask

- 100 g of fresh horse sorrel root

- 1 teaspoon of glycerin

- Birch leaves tincture

- Lemon juice

Grate 100 g of fresh horse sorrel root on a small grater, mix with 1 teaspoon of glycerin and apply to the skin of your face. Leave the mask for 10-15 minutes. Wash it off with a strong tincture of birch leaves acidified with lemon juice. Then apply cream to your face. This mask has a strong astringent effect and is recommended for oily skin with enlarged pores.

✔ **Calendula mask**

- Calendula tincture (20 g of flowers, 100 ml of vodka)

- 100 ml of water

Dilute 1 teaspoon of calendula tincture (for its preparation take 20 g of flowers and leave to infuse for two weeks in 100 ml of vodka) with 100 ml of warm water. Moisten a gauze napkin and put the mask on your face and leave for 15 minutes. The mask has an antiseptic and astringent effect.

✔ **Yoghurt and egg white mask**

- 1 egg white

- 100 g of natural yoghurt

Mix 1 egg white and 100 g of natural yoghurt. Apply to your face and wash off in 15-20 minutes. This mask narrows pores, improving complexion and skin surface.

✔ **Tomato mask**

- 1 tomato

Put slices of a tomato on your face and leave for 25-30 minutes. Wash them off, at first with warm and then with cold water. It is recommended for oily skin of sallow complexion with large pores.

✔ **Honey mask with egg white and flour**

- 1 egg white

- 1 teaspoon of honey

- Flour

Add 1 teaspoon of honey into a whipped egg white little-by-little, stir, then thicken it with flour to the consistency of gruel. Apply the mask to your face and leave for 20 minutes.

✔ Egg mask with green tea

- 1 egg white

- 3-5 drops of lemon juice

- 1 teaspoon of strong green tea

- 1-2 teaspoons of bran or ground oat flakes

Whip the egg white into froth with a whisk or a mixer. Add 3-5 drops of lemon juice and 1 teaspoon of strong green tea. It is possible to add 1-2 teaspoons of bran or ground oat flakes to make the mixture thicker. Apply the mask for 25-30 minutes, wash it off with warm, and then with cool water. Then apply cream to your face.

✔ Apricot with egg white

- 1 apricot

- 1 egg white

Mix the pulp of an apricot with a whipped egg white and apply to the skin of your face.

Nourishing masks for oily facial skin

✔ Yeast mask

- 10 g of yeast

- 2 tablespoons of warm milk

- 1 egg yolk

- Lemon juice

- Rye flour

Break 10 g of yeast in 2 tablespoons of warm milk, add the egg yolk and several drops of lemon juice. Stir to the consistency of gruel, adding rye flour to the mix. Put the mask on your face for 20 minutes. Wash it off with warm, then with cool water.

✔ Aloe mask with honey

- 2 teaspoons of biostimulating aloe juice

- 4 teaspoons of liquid honey

Mix 2 teaspoons of biostimulating aloe juice with 4 teaspoons of liquid honey. Put this mixture on the skin of your face and leave for 10-15 minutes. Then wash it off with soft warm water.

✔ Curd-honey mask

- 2 tablespoons of low-fat curds

- 1 teaspoon of honey

- 1 egg

Mix 2 tablespoons of low-fat curds with 1 teaspoon of honey and half of a whipped egg. Leave the mask on your skin for 20 minutes, wash it off with warm water, then rinse the face with cold water. This mask moistens and nourishes skin.

✔ Curd-carrot mask

- 1 teaspoon of low-fat curds

- 1 teaspoon of milk

- 1 teaspoon of carrot juice

- 1 teaspoon of olive or corn oil

Mix the low-fat curds, fresh milk, carrot juice and olive or corn oil. Apply this mixture to the skin of your face and leave for 15-20 minutes. Wash it off with warm, then with cool water.

✔ Kefir-honey mask

- 2 tablespoons of low-fat kefir

- 1 teaspoon of honey

- Half a teaspoon of lemon juice

Mix 2 tablespoons of low-fat kefir with 1 teaspoon of honey and add half a teaspoon of lemon juice. Leave the mask on your face for 15-20 minutes, then wash it off with warm water.

✔ Creamy-peach mask

- 1 ripe peach

- 3-4 strawberries

- 1 tablespoon of low-fat cream

- 1 tablespoon of rose water

Mash and mix the pulp of the peach and the strawberries, add 1 tablespoon of low-fat cream and 1 tablespoon of rose water. Stir carefully and apply the mask to your face. Leave it for 15 minutes, then wash it off with cool water.

✔ Honey-orange mask

- 1 orange

- Honey

Squeeze the juice out of the orange and cool it. Put a thin layer of preheated honey on your clean and dry skin upon your face and neck. In 15 minutes remove the honey with a cotton wool ball moistened in cold orange juice, and then wipe your skin well with the same juice. The mask promotes skin nourishment and makes it healthy.

✔ Cabbage mask

- Fresh cabbage leaves

- 1 egg white

Chop the cabbage leaves, mix with a whipped egg white and put this mixture on the skin of your face. Leave the mask for 20 minutes, then wash it off with cool water.

✔ Pea mask

- 2 tablespoons of fresh green peas, mashed
- 1 tablespoon of low-fat cream

Mix 2 tablespoons of fresh green peas (mashed) with 1 tablespoon of low-fat cream. Put the mask on your face and leave it for 15-20 minutes, then wash it off with cool water.

✔ Beet mask 1

- Beet
- Natural low-fat yoghurt
- 1 egg yolk

Mix 1 tablespoon of fresh beet grated on a small grater with 1 tablespoon of natural low-fat yoghurt and egg yolk. Apply this mixture to your face and leave it for 20 minutes. Wash the mask off with warm water.

✔ Beet mask 2

- Boiled beet
- 1 aloe leaf
- 1 tablespoon of low-fat curds
- 1 tablespoon of tutsan extract (1.5 tablespoons of tutsan herb per 200 ml of water)

Mix 2 tablespoons of boiled beet grated on a small grater with 1 teaspoon of well-crushed aloe leaf, 1 tablespoon of low-fat curds and 1 tablespoon of tutsan extract. Apply the mask for 10-15 minutes, then wash it off with warm water.

✔ Carrot mask

- Medium carrot
- 1 egg white
- 1 tablespoon of rye flour

Grate one average carrot on a small plastic grater and mix with a whipped egg white and 1 tablespoon of rye flour. Apply this mixture to the skin of your face for 15-20 minutes, then wash it off with cool water. The mask nourishes, freshens and vitaminizes skin.

✔ Pumpkin mask

- 2 tablespoons of boiled pumpkin
- 2 teaspoons of olive oil

Mash 2 tablespoons of boiled pumpkin well, adding 2 teaspoons of olive oil and apply the mixture to the skin of your face. Leave the mask for 20 minutes, then wash it off with cool water.

✔ Peach mask

- Peaches
- 1 tablespoon of oat meal

Mash the peaches and mix 2 tablespoons of peach pulp with 1 tablespoon of oatmeal. Put this mixture on the skin of your face, leave for 15 minutes, then wash it off with warm water and rinse your face with cool water. The mask nourishes, moistens and softens skin.

✔ Grapes mask

- 5-6 grapes
- 1 egg yolk
- 1 teaspoon of starch

Mash 5-6 grapes and mix with the egg yolk and 1 teaspoon of starch. Put this mixture on your face, leave for 20 minutes and wash it off with warm, then with cool water. This mask nourishes skin well.

✓ **Strawberry-honey mask**

- 3-4 large strawberries

- 1 teaspoon of honey

Mash 3-4 large strawberries and mix with 1 teaspoon of honey. Apply this mask to your face and leave for 10 minutes, then wash it off with cool water.

✓ **Raspberry mask**

- 2 tablespoons of raspberries, mashed

- 1 teaspoon of curdled milk

Mix 2 tablespoons of mashed raspberries with 1 teaspoon of curdled milk and apply this paste to the skin of your face. Leave the mask for 10-15 minutes and wash it off with cool water. This nourishing mask also clears and moistens skin.

✓ **Cranberry mask**

- Cranberries or cranberry juice

Moisten a gauze napkin in cranberry juice and apply to your face and neck for 15 minutes. In the case of a burning sensation, dilute the juice with water at a 1:2 or 1:3 ratio. Using mashed berries is also an option. Wash the mask off with cold water, then apply low-fat sour cream to your face. This procedure is to be carried out 2-3 times a week. This mask not only nourishes but also bleaches skin.

✓ **Yoghurt mask with herbs**

- 2 tablespoons of dandelion, sage, plantain or rosemary leaves

- 2 tablespoons of natural low-fat yoghurt

- Wheat sprouts, crushed

Mix 2 tablespoons of crushed dandelion, sage, plantain or rosemary leaves with 2 tablespoons of natural low-fat yoghurt and add crushed wheat sprouts to the consistency of thick gruel. Put the mask on your face and leave for 10 minutes. Wash it off, at first with warm then with cool water.

✓ Mask with olive oil

- 1 egg yolk

- 1 tablespoon of honey

- 1 tablespoon of olive oil

- Half a cup of oat flakes

Mix the egg yolk and 1 tablespoon of honey. Add 1 tablespoon of olive oil and half a cup of oat flakes. Apply the mask to your face and leave for 15-20 minutes. Wash it off with warm water.

✓ Plum mask

- 1 ripe plum

- 1 egg white

Peel and mash 1 ripe plum, add a whipped egg white and apply to your skin for 20 minutes. Wash it off with warm water.

✓ Sorrel leaf mask

- 3-5 sorrel leaves

- 2 tablespoons of low-fat curds

- Sour milk

Take 3-5 sorrel leaves, cut them with a knife into small pieces, mash with a wooden spoon and mix with 2 tablespoons of low-fat curds. Apply the mask for 20 minutes, then remove it with paper napkins and wipe your face with sour milk. The mask nourishes, strengthens skin and makes it healthy.

Toning masks for oily facial skin

✔ **Curd-salt mask**

- 1 tablespoon of fresh curds

- 2 tablespoons of kefir

- Half a teaspoon of lemon juice

- 1 teaspoon of table salt

Mix 1 tablespoon of fresh curds with 2 tablespoons of kefir. Add half a teaspoon of lemon juice and 1 teaspoon of table salt. Stir well. Put this mask on your face and leave for 20 minutes, then wash it off with warm water and rinse with cold water.

✔ **Yeast mask with onion juice**

- 10 g of yeast

- 1 tablespoon of onion juice

- 1 teaspoon of honey

Break 10 g of yeast in 1 tablespoon of onion juice and add 1 teaspoon of honey. Stir this mixture well and apply to the skin of your face. Leave the mask for 15 minutes. Wash it off at first with warm, then with cool water.

✔ **Flower mask with aloe juice**

- 1 tablespoon of aloe juice

- 1 tablespoon of rose petals

- Half a tablespoon of linden flowers

- 1 tablespoon of chamomile flowers

- Half a tablespoon of peppermint leaves

- Half a tablespoon of sage leaves

- Non-greasy nourishing cream

Mix 1 tablespoon of aloe juice with the crushed fresh leaves and flowers: 1 tablespoon of rose petals, half a tablespoon of linden flowers, 1 tablespoon of chamomile flowers, half a tablespoon of peppermint leaves and half a tablespoon of sage leaves. Apply this mixture to the skin of your face, having first applied a non-greasy nourishing cream. Leave the mask for 15 minutes, then wash it off with warm water.

✔ Mask with green tea

- 3 tablespoons of green tea

- 2 tablespoons of curdled milk, low-fat kefir or natural yoghurt

Grind 3 tablespoons of green tea well and mix with 2 tablespoons of curdled milk, low-fat kefir or natural yoghurt. Put the mask on the skin of your face and leave for 15 minutes. Wash it off with warm, then with cool water. Green tea tones facial skin well, making it elastic and resilient.

✔ Mask with viburnum juice

- 1 egg white

- 1 teaspoon of curdled milk

- 1 teaspoon of honey

- 3-4 spoons of oat flakes

- 1 tablespoon of viburnum juice

Whip the egg white with 1 teaspoon of curdled milk and 1 teaspoon of honey, add 3-4 spoons of oat flakes and 1 tablespoon of viburnum juice. Stir carefully and apply the mixture to the skin of your face. Wash the mask off after 15-20 minutes with warm water. It is recommended that you apply the mask 1-2 times a week.

✓ **Mask with herbs 1**

- 2 tablespoons of fresh peppermint leaves

- 2 tablespoons of fresh plantain leaves

- 2 tablespoons of fresh melissa leaves

- 2 tablespoons of fresh nettle leaves

- 2 tablespoons of fresh yarrow leaves

- 1 tablespoon of fresh low-fat curds

- 1 tablespoon of kefir

Mix 2 tablespoons of finely crushed fresh peppermint, plantain, melissa, nettle and yarrow leaves with 1 tablespoon of fresh low-fat curds and 1 tablespoon of kefir. Apply the mixture to the skin of your face for 20 minutes. Wash it off with warm water and wipe the face with a cube of mint ice.

✓ **Mask with herbs 2**

- Hawthorn flowers

- Caseweed herb

- Sage herb

- Dandelion roots

- 200 ml of water

- 2 tablespoons of fresh curds

Mix the hawthorn blossom, caseweed herb, sage herb and dandelion roots in equal parts. Add 1 tablespoon of this mixture to 200 ml of water, heat on a water bath for 15 minutes, let it infuse for 45 minutes and filter. Mix 2 tablespoons of herbal tincture with 2 tablespoons of fresh curds and apply the mask to your face. Leave it for 20 minutes, then wash it off with cool water.

✓ **Mask with herbs 3**

- 1 tablespoon of calendula flowers

- 1 tablespoon of tutsan herb

- 1 tablespoon of yarrow herb

- 1 tablespoon of plantain leaves

- Boiling water

Crush 1 tablespoon of calendula flowers, tutsan herb, yarrow herb and plantain leaves. Add boiling water untill the mixture has the consistency of thick gruel. Apply the paste to the skin of your face and cover with a gauze napkin. Leave for 15-20 minutes, then wash it off with warm water. This vitamin mask tones skin very well.

Creams and ointments for oily facial skin

✔ Cucumber cream

- 50 g of day-time cream for oily skin

- 8 teaspoons of cucumber juice

Add 50 g of any day-time cream for oily skin to 8 teaspoons of cucumber juice and stir well. Keep the prepared cream in a refrigerator. Good for bleaching skin.

✔ Lemon cream with aloe

- 30 g of a non-greasy nourishing cream

- 1/3 of teaspoon of lemon juice

- 1 aloe leaf

Add 1/3 of teaspoon of lemon juice and 1/3 of teaspoon of well-crushed aloe leaf to 30 g of non-greasy nourishing cream and stir carefully. Spread a thin layer of the cream upon your face. In a few minutes remove the remains with a napkin or a cotton wool ball. This is a good way of cleansing oily skin.

✔ Sea-buckthorn cream

- 50 g of fresh butter

- 1 tablespoon of mashed sea-buckthorn berries

- Lemon juice

Melt 50 g of fresh butter on a water bath, then cool it a little. Add 1 tablespoon of mashed sea-buckthorn berries, 10 drops of lemon juice and stir well. Keep the prepared cream in a refrigerator. Apply this cream to your face for the night.

✔ Cream with viburnum juice

- 40 ml of a non-greasy nourishing cream

- 1 teaspoon of viburnum juice

Add 1 teaspoon of viburnum juice to 40 ml of a non-greasy nourishing cream little-by-little while stirring well. The cream possesses bleaching properties. It is better to apply it for the night. Keep this cream in a refrigerator.

✔ Cream with apricot kernel oil

- 10 g of white beeswax

- 40 ml of apricot kernel oil

- 2 teaspoons of rose water

- 4-5 drops of rose oil

Melt 10 g of white beeswax on a water bath, add 40 ml of apricot kernel oil, 2 teaspoons of rose water and stir well. Let it cool down and add 4-5 drops of rose oil.

Use as a night-time cream.

Skin care recipes for dry facial skin

Dry facial skin (p.88)

Washing, purifying for dry facial skin (p.89)

Cleansing masks for dry facial skin (p.93)

Moisturizing, freshening masks for dry facial skin (p.96)

Softening masks for dry facial skin (p.101)

Nourishing vitamin masks for dry facial skin (p.107)

Creams, oils and ointments for dry facial skin (p.119)

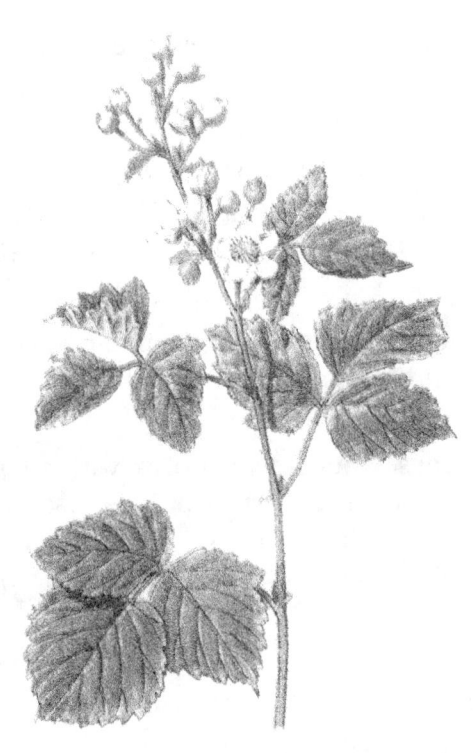

Dry facial skin

Dry skin can have various origins.

As such, its appearance differs. In youth and middle age groups, the dryness can be "natural".

In this case, dry skin looks gentle, thin and with a matte tone. Pores are unnoticeable, but tiny wrinkles may appear even at a young age.

If not taken proper care of, dry skin might peel, shrink or grow irritated.

Such skin reacts badly to changes in temperature, washing with soap, ointments and some softening creams.

Dry skin is very sensitive to adverse influences. It is deprived of shine, frequently peels, loses elasticity quickly and wrinkles appear rather early.

The main action to undertake for dry skin is regular nourishing and moisturizing, protection against sunlight. Cleanse dry skin twice a day.

In the morning cleanse your face and neck with a liquid cream, vegetable oil or toilet milk. Then wipe your face with toning linden flower, marshmallow root or linseed tincture. Apply cream and in 15-20 minutes remove the surplus with a paper napkin.

In the evening cleanse your face with a cosmetic milk or cream. After cleansing apply some greasy nourishing vitamin cream.

Nourishing and moisturizing masks are necessary for dry skin twice a week.

Washing, purifying for dry facial skin

✔ Oat flakes

- 1-2 tablespoons of oat flakes

- Boiling water

Pour boiling water over 1-2 tablespoons of oat flakes and leave to infuse a little. Apply the warm mass to your face with light circular movements. Then wash it off with soft water.

✔ Almond bran

- 1 tablespoon of almond bran

- Hot water

Mix 1 tablespoon of almond bran with a bit of hot water to the consistency of gruel. Apply this mask to your face and leave for 10-15 minutes, then wash it off with warm water.

✔ Rice bran

- Half a glass of rice bran

- Warm water

Add warm water to half a glass of rice bran and stir to the consistency of gruel. Apply a thick layer of this mass to the skin of your face and leave for 10 minutes. Then massage the face a little and rinse with warm water. This cleansing procedure makes skin soft and elastic.

✔ Melon for dry skin

- 1 melon

Peel a melon, mash slices with a fork or grate them and wring the juice out. Wipe the skin of your face with a cotton wool ball moistened in the juice.

✔ Almond toilet water

- 50 g of peeled sweet almonds
- Half a liter of water
- 5 g of grated children's soap

Crush 50 g of peeled sweet almonds in a mortar, add half a liter of water, let it infuse for a day, filter it and wring the mass out. Then add 5 g of grated soap and mix until it dissolves. This almond water is suitable for a gentle dry skin.

✔ Cucumber milk

- 100 ml of fresh milk
- 1 cucumber

Leave several slices of cucumber in 100 ml of fresh milk for half an hour, then filter this milk and use for wiping dry skin. It can be stored in a refrigerator for no more than 2-3 days.

✔ Mint extract for face washing

- 1-2 tablespoons of peppermint
- 400 ml of hot water

Peppermint extract is recommended for washing the face in the case of dry skin. Add 1-2 tablespoons of peppermint to 400 ml of hot water, boil on a low heat for 5-10 minutes, then cool and filter.

✔ Yolk-cream lotion

- 1 egg yolk
- 100 ml of cream
- 1 teaspoon of lemon juice
- 1 teaspoon of onion juice
- 1 tablespoon of vodka

Mix 1 egg yolk with about 100 ml of cream and add 1 teaspoon of lemon juice, 1 teaspoon of onion juice and 1 tablespoon of vodka. Wipe your face with this lotion and wash it off with warm water after 30 minutes.

✔ Yolk-lemon lotion

- 1 egg yolk

- 2 tablespoons of olive or almond oil

- 2 tablespoons of cognac

- Lemon juice (1/2 of lemon)

Whip 1 egg yolk with 2 tablespoons of olive or almond oil, add 2 tablespoons of cognac and lemon juice. Mix well and wipe the skin of your face. In two to three minutes rinse the face with warm water.

✔ Cucumber lotion

- 1 small fresh cucumber

- Vodka

- Water

- Glycerin

Grate a small fresh cucumber on a grater and add an equal volume of vodka. Infuse in a dark place for two weeks, filter, dilute with water 1:1 and add 1 teaspoon of glycerin per 100 ml of the lotion. This lotion possesses bleaching action.

✔ Grapefruit lotion

- Grapefruit juice (1 big grapefruit)

- 2 tablespoons of vodka

- 1 egg yolk

- 100 ml of fresh cream

Mix grapefruit juice with 2 tablespoons of vodka. Whip 1 egg yolk with about 100 ml of fresh cream in a separate pan. Blend both mixtures and pour in a bottle. Shake well before usage. This lotion can be kept in a refrigerator for five days.

✔ Melon lotion

- Melon juice

- Milk

- Mineral water

Mix in equal parts melon juice, milk and mineral water. Wipe your face with the lotion every morning. It cleanses, nourishes and tones the skin.

✔ Lotion with linden flowers

- 1 tablespoon of linden flowers

- 100 ml of boiling water

- 1 teaspoon of honey

- 2-3 drops of lemon juice

Add 1 tablespoon of linden flowers to 100 ml of boiling water, heat on a water bath for 15 minutes, let it infuse for 45 minutes, filter and add 1 teaspoon of honey and 2-3 drops of lemon juice. Wipe your face carefully.

✔ Mint lotion

- 1 tablespoon of peppermint

- 200 ml of boiling water

- 1 teaspoon of glycerin

Add 1 tablespoon of peppermint to 200 ml of boiling water and let it infuse in a closed vessel for 30 minutes. Then filter, add 1 teaspoon of glycerin and wipe the skin of your face with the lotion.

✔ Anise lotion

- 1 teaspoon of crushed anise fruits

- 100 ml of boiling water

Add 1 teaspoon of crushed anise fruits to 100 ml of boiling water, infuse until it cools, filter and use for cleansing the skin of your face. This lotion softens and smoothes dry skin.

✔ Rose lotion

- 3 glasses of red rose petals

- Almond or peach oil

Add 3 glasses of red roses petals to the almond or peach oil so that the oil covers them whole. Heat on a water bath until the petals fully lose their color. Wipe your face with this lotion several times a day. This lotion has a great toning effect.

Cleansing masks for dry facial skin

✔ Oatmeal mask

- 3 tablespoons of oatmeal

- 1 teaspoon of honey

- 1 tablespoon of vegetable oil

- 3 tablespoons of milk

Mix carefully 1 teaspoon of honey, 1 tablespoon of vegetable oil, 3 tablespoons of milk and 3 tablespoons of oatmeal. Apply the mixture to the skin of your face and wash it off with warm water after 20 minutes.

✔ Tomato mask

- Tomato juice (1-2 tomatoes)

- 1 egg yolk

- 1 tablespoon of oatmeal

Mix the tomato juice with 1 egg yolk and 1 tablespoon of oatmeal. Put the mask on your face and leave for 20 minutes. Wash it off with warm soft water.

✓ **Tomato mask 2**

- 1 tomato

- Potato starch

- Half a teaspoon of olive, sesame or sunflower oil

Grate a tomato on a plastic grater and mix with the potato starch until you get gruel. Add half a teaspoon of olive, sesame or sunflower oil and put this mixture on the skin of your face. Leave the mask for 20 minutes, wash it off with warm water and then rinse your face with cold.

✓ **Tomato mask 3**

- 1 tomato

- 2 tablespoons of curds

- 1 teaspoon of cream

- 1 teaspoon of sunflower oil or wheat sprout oil

Chop 1 tomato and mix with 2 tablespoons of curds, 1 teaspoon of cream and 1 teaspoon of sunflower oil or wheat sprout oil. Leave the mask on your face for 20 minutes, then wash it off with warm water and rinse your face with cold water.

✓ **Corn mask**

- 2 tablespoons of corn flour

- Warm water

Blend 2 tablespoons of corn flour with warm water to the consistency of gruel and apply the mask to your face. Wash it off with cool water after 10 minutes and apply a nourishing cream.

✔ Carrot mask

- Large carrot

Grate 1 large carrot on a small plastic grater, wring the juice out, moisten a gauze napkin in it and apply to your face and leave for 20-30 minutes. This mask clears and softens dry skin.

✔ Wild strawberry mask

- Half a glass of wild strawberries

- Half a teaspoon of glycerin

- Cool water

Mash half a glass of wild strawberries, add half a teaspoon of glycerin. Add some cool water and stir. Put this mixture on your face and leave for 15 minutes, then wash it off with warm water. This mask clears and tones skin.

✔ Grape mask

- Grapes

Wring out 4-5 spoonfuls of grape juice, moisten a gauze or linen napkin in it and apply to your face. Leave the mask for 15 minutes, then wash it off with warm water and apply a nourishing cream. The grape mask clears and tones skin well, making it elastic and velvety.

✔ Almond mask

- 1 tablespoon of peeled ground almonds

- 1 tablespoon of fresh cream

Mix 1 tablespoon of peeled ground almonds with 1 tablespoon of fresh cream. Put the mixture on the skin of your face for 15 minutes. Wash it off with warm water. This mask has a clearing and peeling effect.

✓ Honey-lemon mask

- 1 tablespoon of honey

- 5-10 drops of lemon juice

- Quarter of a teaspoon of oat flour

Mix the lemon juice, honey and the fourth part of a teaspoon of oat flour. Blend thoroughly. Apply the mask to the cleansed skin of your face for 15 minutes, then wash it off with cool water or remove with the help of lemon lotion or tincture.

Moisturizing, freshening masks for dry facial skin

✓ Curd mask

- 4 teaspoons of fat curds

- 1 teaspoon of honey

Mix 4 teaspoons of fat curds with 1 teaspoon of honey. Apply the mask for 20 minutes, then wash it off with warm water and apply some moisturizing cream to your face.

✓ Sour cream mask with grapefruit

- 1 tablespoon of sour cream

- Half a tablespoon of honey

- Half a teaspoon of grated grapefruit rind

Add half a teaspoon of grated grapefruit rind to 1 tablespoon of sour cream and half tablespoon of honey. Stir well and apply the mixture to the skin of your face. Leave the mask for 15-20 minutes. Wash it off with cool water or cold tea. This mask moistens, tones and smoothes skin.

✓ Cucumber mask

- 1 cucumber

- 2 tablespoons of fresh milk

Peel and grate the cucumber on a small plastic grater, add 2 tablespoons of fresh milk and put the mask on your face for 15 minutes. Wash it off with warm water. The mask is recommended for very dry skin.

✔ Marrow mask 1

- 1 marrow squash

Peel and grate the marrow on a small plastic grater, spread the received mask on a gauze or linen napkin and apply to your face. Leave the mask for 15 minutes, then wash it off with warm water.

✔ Marrow mask 2

- 1 marrow squash

- Fresh milk

Put thin slices of raw marrow on your face and in 20 minutes remove them and wipe your skin with fresh milk. Marrow squash not only moistens but also clears and tones skin.

✔ Potato mask 1

- 1-2 potatoes

Peel and grate 1-2 fresh potatoes on a small plastic grater and put the potato mask on your face and leave for 15-20 minutes. Then wash it off with warm, then with cool water. This mask moistens, clears and smoothes skin well.

✔ Potato mask 2

- Potatoes boiled in their skins

- Half a teaspoon of lemon juice

Peel and mash the potatoes boiled in their skins, mix with half a teaspoon of lemon juice and put on your face for 15-20 minutes. Wash it off with warm, then with cool water. This mask freshens and smoothes skin.

✓ **Pumpkin mask**

- 2 tablespoons of boiled pumpkin pulp

- 1 tablespoon of olive or any other vegetable oil

Blend 2 tablespoons of boiled pumpkin pulp with 1 tablespoon of olive or any other vegetable oil and put the mixture on the skin of your face. Leave the mask for 15 minutes, then wash it off with warm water. Pumpkin masks clear, moisten and tone skin.

✓ **Apple mask**

- 1 apple

- 1 tablespoon of olive oil

Mix 2 tablespoons of apple grated on a small plastic grater with 1 tablespoon of olive oil and put this mixture on the skin of your face. Leave the mask for 10-15 minutes, then wash it off with warm water.

✓ **Strawberry mask**

- 100-150 g of strawberries

- 1 tablespoon of creamy natural yoghurt

Mash 100-150 g of strawberries, mix with 1 tablespoon of creamy natural yoghurt and put this paste on your face. Leave the mask for 10 minutes. Wash it off with warm water.

✓ **Currant mask**

- 1 tablespoon of black currant juice

- Wheat bran

Mix 1 tablespoon of black currant juice with the wheat bran to the consistency of cream. Apply this mixture to the skin of your face for 10-15 minutes and wash it off with cool water. This mask moistens and tones skin well.

✔ Grape mask

- 1 teaspoon of curds
- 1 teaspoon of honey
- 2 teaspoons of grape juice

Blend 1 teaspoon of curds with 1 teaspoon of honey and add 2 teaspoons of grape juice. Put this mixture on your face and leave for 10-15 minutes, wash it off with cool water. This mask is useful for thin sensitive skin.

✔ Herbal tincture mask

- Chamomile flowers
- Linden flowers
- Rose petals
- Peppermint leaves
- 200 ml of water

Mix 2 parts of chamomile flowers, 2 parts of linden flowers, 1 part of rose petals and 1 part of peppermint leaves. Add 2 tablespoons of this mixture to 200 ml of water, heat on a water bath for 15 minutes, let it infuse for 45 minutes and filter. Moisten a gauze napkin in this tincture and apply to your face for 15 minutes.

✔ Aubergine (eggplant) mask

- 1 aubergine (eggplant)
- Milk or mineral water

Put thin strips of aubergine (eggplant) on your face (excluding area around the eyes), cover with a napkin or gauze. In 10 minutes remove the strips and rinse the face with milk or mineral water.

✔ Aloe and cucumber mask

- 1 cucumber

- 1 tablespoon of mashed aloe

- 1 tablespoon of tutsan extract

- 1 teaspoon of vegetable oil

Grate a cucumber on a small grater, add 1 tablespoon of mashed aloe, 1 tablespoon of tutsan extract and 1 teaspoon of vegetable oil. Blend all the ingredients thoroughly. Put an even layer of this mixture on your face, excluding the area of the eyelids. In 25-30 minutes wash it off with warm water and apply a moisturizing cream.

✔ Mint decoction mask

- Peppermint leaves (fresh or dried)

- Water

Add crushed peppermint leaves to water at a 1:3 ratio, bring to a boil, boil for 2-3 minutes, cool it a little and spread a thin layer of the warm mixture on a gauze napkin. Apply to your face for 15-20 minutes, then remove and rinse the face with warm water. Repeat this procedure every other day for three weeks.

✔ Milk and honey mask

- 2 tablespoons of flour

- 3 tablespoons of milk

- 1 teaspoon of honey

- 2 tablespoons of grated apple

Blend 2 tablespoons of flour, 3 tablespoons of milk, 1 teaspoon of honey and 2 tablespoons of grated apple until you get a thick gruel and apply to your skin for 15-20 minutes.

Softening masks for dry facial skin

✓ Oil mask

- Sunflower or olive oil

- Dry skin lotion

Moisten two to three layers of gauze in warmed sunflower or olive oil and apply to your face and neck for 10-15 minutes. After this procedure wipe the face with lotion for dry skin. This mask is recommended for very dry skin.

✓ Yolk-oil mask

- Olive, peach or almond oil

- 1 egg yolk

- Water

Cleanse the face with a cotton wool ball moistened in olive, peach or almond oil. Then grease the skin with the resulting oil, apply the egg yolk and periodically moistening fingers with hot water spread it until a white foamy mask is formed. Leave this mask for 15-20 minutes, then wash it off. It is very useful against dry skin that peels.

✓ Honey mask with rose water

- 1 tablespoon of honey

- Rose water

Mix 1 tablespoon of honey with about half a tablespoon of rose water. Put this mixture on the skin of your face and leave for 15-

20 minutes. Then wash it off with warm water and wipe with rose water.

✔ Mask with honey

- 1 teaspoon of honey
- 1 egg yolk
- 1 tablespoon of cream
- Rose infusion

Blend the honey, egg yolk and cream until the mixture becomes white.

Apply this mixture to your face and neck for 20 minutes. Wash the mask off with warm water, and then rinse the face with cooled rose infusion. (To prepare the infusion, add the leaves of two rose buds to a glass of boiling water, infuse it for 3 hours, then filter and cool in a refrigerator.)

✔ Cucumber-honey mask

- 3 tablespoons of honey
- Half teaspoon of lemon juice
- 1 cucumber

Mix 3 tablespoons of honey with half a teaspoon of lemon juice. Put this mixture on the facial skin and massage it for 5 minutes with light movements. Then place slices of a fresh cucumber on the face and leave the mask for 15 minutes. Wash it off with warm, then with cool water.

✔ Potato mask

- 1 large potato boiled (skin on)
- 1 egg yolk
- Hot milk

Peel and mash one large potato, add 1 egg yolk and some hot milk, blend well. Apply the mask to your face while it's warm. Leave for 15-20 minutes then wash it off first with warm, then with cool water. This mask softens and calms skin, smoothing it.

✔ Almond mask

- 1 glass of peeled almonds

- 400 ml of boiling water

- 2 tablespoons of lemon juice

- 2 tablespoons of distilled water

Add one glass of peeled almonds to 400 ml of boiling water. After 5 minutes pour the water away, mince the almonds and add 2 tablespoons of lemon juice and 2 tablespoons of distilled water. Stir carefully and apply the mask to your face. Leave for 20 minutes, then wash it off with warm water and apply some cream for dry skin. This mask softens skin and removes inflammations.

✔ Oatmeal mask 1

- 1 tablespoon of oatmeal

- 1 tablespoon of greasy cream

Mix 1 tablespoon of oatmeal with 1 tablespoon of greasy cream and apply the mixture to the skin of your face with light massaging movements. Leave the mask for 20 minutes, then wash it off with warm water and rinse with cool water. This mask is useful for especially sensitive skin that is prone to allergic reactions.

✔ Oatmeal mask 2

- 1 egg yolk

- 1 tablespoon of oatmeal

Mix 1 egg yolk with 1 tablespoon of oatmeal and apply the mixture to your face. Leave the mask for 15-20 minutes, then wash it off with warm water. This mask softens and calms gentle sensitive skin.

✓ **Oatmeal mask 3**

- 2 tablespoons of oatmeal

- Warm water

- 1 tablespoon of sea-buckthorn juice

Blend 2 tablespoons of oatmeal with warm water to the consistency of thick gruel and add 1 tablespoon of sea-buckthorn juice. Leave the mask for 20 minutes, wash it off with warm water and rinse the face with cool water. This mask softens and nourishes skin well.

✓ **Linseed mask**

- 1 teaspoon of linseed

- 400 ml of water

Add 1 teaspoon of linseed to 400 ml of water and cook on a low heat until the seeds begin to boil softly. Let the mixture cool down a little and apply it to your face. Leave the mask for 20 minutes. Wash it off first with warm, then with cold water. This mask softens skin well and prevents inflammation. It is especially useful in cold weather. A course of 10-15 procedures (2-3 masks a week) is necessary to protect skin from the cold.

✓ **Linseed mask with herbs**

- Fresh thyme leaves

- Fresh mint leaves

- Fresh melissa leaves

- Fresh common mallow (Malva sylvestris) leaves

- 1 tablespoon of linseed flour

- 400 ml of boiling water

Mix chopped fresh thyme, mint, melissa and common mallow leaves in equal parts. Add 2 tablespoons of this mixture and 1 tablespoon of linseed flour to 200 ml of boiled water, stir and let it cool down. Apply the mask to your face for 20 minutes, then wash it off with warm water and rinse the face with cold water.

✔ Coltsfoot mask

- Fresh coltsfoot leaves

- Milk

Add fresh milk to 2 tablespoons of well crushed fresh coltsfoot leaves and stir to the consistency of gruel. Apply the mixture to your face, leave for 20 minutes, then wash it off with cool water. This mask helps skin in dry weather.

✔ Green mask

- Fresh sea-buckthorn leaves

- Fresh melissa leaves

- Fresh raspberry leaves

- 50 ml of boiling water

- Oatmeal

Mix fresh sea-buckthorn, melissa and raspberry leaves in equal parts. Add 1 teaspoon of this crushed mixture to 50 ml of boiling water and stir, adding oatmeal until you get a thick gruel. Cool the mixture and apply it to your face. Leave for 20 minutes, then wash it off with cool water. This mask softens skin, eliminating peeling.

✔ Grapefruit mask

- 1 egg yolk

- 1 tablespoon of grapefruit juice

- 1 teaspoon of vegetable oil

- 1 tablespoon of sour cream

- Crumb of black bread

- Milk

Add 1 tablespoon grapefruit juice and 1 teaspoon of vegetable oil to a kneaded egg yolk, whip everything and add a tablespoon of sour cream. To make the mixture thicker you can add the crumb of black bread soaked in milk. Apply this mixture to your face for 15-20 minutes, then wash it off and spread your skin with cream. After 10 minutes remove the remaining cream with a paper napkin.

✔ **Yolk and green tea mask**

- 1 egg yolk

- 1-2 teaspoons of olive mayonnaise

- Half a teaspoon of green tea

Knead 1 egg yolk with 1-2 teaspoons of olive mayonnaise and mix with half a teaspoon of small-leaved green tea (you can grind green tea in a mortar or in a coffee grinder). Put the mask on your face and wash it off with warm water after 20-25 minutes. After removing the mask apply a moisturizing cream.

✔ **Egg-apricot mask**

- 1 egg yolk

- 1 teaspoon of apricot oil

Mix 1 egg yolk with 1 teaspoon of apricot oil. Apply the mask to your face with rubbing movements.

✔ **Lemon mask**

- Half a lemon

- 1 egg yolk

- 1 tablespoon of ground germinating corn seeds

- 1 teaspoon of honey

Mix lemon, a whipped yolk, 1 tablespoon of ground germinating corn seeds and 1 teaspoon of honey. Apply the mask for 45 minutes. Remove it and wash your face with warm milk. This mask helps skin become soft, elastic and smooth.

✓ **Salad mask**

- 1 tablespoon of salad leaves

- 1 tablespoon of sour cream

- Half a teaspoon of olive oil

Mix 1 tablespoon of salad leaves mashed into gruel with 1 tablespoon of sour cream, add half a teaspoon of olive oil and put this mixture on dry skin zones. Leave the mask for 20 minutes, then wash it off with cool water.

Nourishing vitamin masks for dry facial skin

✓ **Curd-yolk mask**

- 1 egg yolk

- 1 teaspoon of curds or cream

Knead 1 egg yolk with 1 teaspoon of fresh curds or cream. Put this mixture on your face for 20 minutes, then wash it off with warm water.

✓ **Curd-strawberry mask**

- 2 teaspoons of curds

- 2 teaspoons of honey

- 2 tablespoons of strawberry juice

Mix 2 teaspoons of curds with 2 teaspoons of honey, add 2 tablespoons of strawberry juice and stir thoroughly. Put a thick layer of this mixture on your face and leave the mask for 10-15 minutes. Wash it off with cool water. This mask is suitable for thin dry sensitive skin.

✔ Curd mask with herbs

- 2 tablespoons of fresh mint leaves
- 2 tablespoons of fresh melissa leaves
- 2 tablespoons of fresh black currant leaves
- 2 tablespoons of fresh nasturtium leaves
- 2 tablespoons of fresh raspberry leaves
- 2 tablespoons of rose petals
- 2 tablespoons of fresh curds
- 1 teaspoon of honey
- Linden flowers or chamomile infusion

Mix 2 tablespoons of well crushed fresh mint, melissa, black currant, nasturtium and raspberry leaves along with rose petals with 2 tablespoons of fresh curds and 1 teaspoon of honey. Put this mixture on your face for 20 minutes, then wash it off with warm water and rinse with cold linden flowers or chamomile infusion.

✔ Milk-carrot mask

- 1 teaspoon of fresh curds
- 1 teaspoon of milk
- 1 teaspoon of olive oil
- 1 teaspoon of carrot juice

Mix 1 teaspoon of fresh curds, milk, olive oil and carrot juice and put this mixture on your face. Leave the mask for 15-20 minutes, then wash it off with soft warm water.

✔ Sour cream mask with carrot juice

- 1 egg yolk
- 1 tablespoon of sour cream
- 1 teaspoon of carrot juice

Mix 1 egg yolk with 1 tablespoon of sour cream and add 1 teaspoon of carrot juice. Put this mixture on your face and leave for 20 minutes. Wash the mask off with warm water.

✔ Honey mask with beer

- 2 tablespoons of unfiltered (live) beer
- 1 teaspoon of wheat sprout oil or olive oil
- 1 tablespoon of honey

Mix 2 tablespoons of unfiltered beer with 1 teaspoon of wheat sprout oil or olive oil, add 1 tablespoon of honey and stir thoroughly. Apply the mixture to your face for 20 minutes, then wash it off with warm water.

✔ Yolk mask with aloe

- 1 egg yolk
- 1 teaspoon of crushed aloe
- 1 tablespoon of sour cream

Mix the egg yolk with 1 teaspoon of aloe and 1 tablespoon of sour cream. Apply this mixture to the skin of your face and neck in layers, each following layer is applied when the previous has dried. Procedure duration: 20-30 minutes. Then wash the mask off with warm water and rinse with cold water.

✔ Yolk-plum mask

- 1 egg yolk
- 1 teaspoon of plum juice

- Linden infusion

Add 1 teaspoon of plum juice to a kneaded yolk. Leave the mask for 20 minutes, then wash it off with warm water and rinse the face with cold linden infusion.

✔ **Yolk-honey mask 1**

- 1 egg yolk

- 1 teaspoon of honey

- 1 teaspoon of glycerin

- Oatmeal

Mix the egg yolk with 1 teaspoon of honey, add 1 teaspoon of glycerin, some oatmeal and stir until you get a consistent texture. Put the mask on your face and leave for 20-30 minutes. Wash it off with warm water and rinse the face with cold water. This nourishing mask prevents the occurrence of wrinkles.

✔ **Yolk-honey mask 2**

- 1 egg yolk

- 1 teaspoon of honey

- 1 teaspoon of olive oil

- Starch or rye flour

Mix the egg yolk with 1 teaspoon of honey, add 1 teaspoon of olive oil and some starch or rye flour to make it thicker. Apply this mixture to your face, leave for 20-30 minutes, then wash it off with cool water. This mask nourishes and softens dry skin well.

✔ **Yolk-onion mask**

- 1 egg yolk

- 1 tablespoon of olive or sesame oil

- 1 tablespoon of onion juice

Whisk the egg yolk, mix with 1 tablespoon of olive or sesame oil, add 1 tablespoon of onion juice, stir well and put this mixture on your face for 10 minutes. Then wash it off with warm water.

✔ Yolk-almond mask

- 1 egg yolk
- 2 tablespoons of sweet almonds
- Toilet water
- Moisturizing cream

Knead 1 egg yolk carefully, adding 2 tablespoons of sweet almonds little-by-little. Apply this mixture to your face for 20 minutes, then remove the mask with a napkin. Wipe the face with toilet water and spread with a moisturizing cream. The mask nourishes and softens skin well, making it elastic.

✔ Yolk mask with quince

- 1 quince
- 1 egg yolk
- 1 tablespoon of olive or almond oil

Peel 1 quince, grate on a small plastic grater and mix with the egg yolk and 1 tablespoon of olive or almond oil. Apply this mixture to your face and leave the mask for 20 minutes. Wash it off with warm, then with cool water.

✔ Yolk-banana mask

- 1 banana
- 1 tablespoon of sour cream
- 1 egg yolk

Mash the pulp of 1 banana carefully, add 1 tablespoon of sour cream and 1 egg yolk and put this mixture on your face. Leave the mask for 10-15 minutes and wash it off with warm water.

✔ Banana-cream mask 1

- Half a banana
- 1 teaspoon of cream

Mash the pulp of half a banana carefully, add 1 teaspoon of cream, stir and put this mask on your face. Wash the mask off with some water after 15 minutes. The mask is useful for dry skin that peels.

✔ Banana-cream mask 2

- 1 ripe banana
- 2 teaspoons of warm cream
- 1 teaspoon of honey

Mix 2 teaspoons of warm cream with 1 teaspoon of honey. Mash 1 ripe banana into pulp and add the cream mixture and honey to it. Apply the mask to your face and neck for 15-20 minutes, then wash it off with warm water.

✔ Carrot mask

- 1 large carrot
- 1 egg yolk
- Half a teaspoon of olive oil

Grate 1 large carrot on a small plastic grater, mix with the egg yolk and half a teaspoon of olive oil. Apply this mixture to your face for 20-30 minutes, then wash it off with warm water.

✔ Beet mask

- 1 fresh beet

- 1 tablespoon of high-fat sour cream

- 1 egg yolk

Mix 1 tablespoon of a fresh beet grated on a small grater with 1 tablespoon of high-fat sour cream and 1 egg yolk. Apply this mixture to your face and leave for 20 minutes, then wash it off with warm water.

✔ Cabbage mask 1

- Cabbage leaves

- 1 egg yolk

- Olive, sunflower or linseed oil

Crush the fresh cabbage into gruel, add the egg yolk and 1 tablespoon of olive, sunflower or linseed oil. Stir thoroughly and apply this mixture to your face and neck for 20 minutes. Wash it off at first with warm, then with cold water. This mask is useful for very dry skin.

✔ Cabbage mask 2

- Cabbage leaf

- Milk

Crush a cabbage leaf, boil it in milk, mash into gruel and apply to your face for 20 minutes. Then wash it off with warm water. This mask nourishes and clears skin.

✔ Marrow squash mask

- 1 egg yolk

- 1 teaspoon of fresh marrow juice

Add 1 teaspoon of fresh marrow juice to a kneaded egg yolk. Apply the mask to your face for 15-20 minutes, then wash it off with warm water.

✔ Apricot mask 1

- Ripe apricots

You can simply slice ripe apricots and put thin slices on your face. The mask is useful for dry, easily irritated skin.

✔ Apricot mask 2

- 2 tablespoons of ripe apricot pulp

- 1 tablespoon of fresh cream

Mix 2 tablespoons of ripe apricot pulp with 1 tablespoon of fresh cream. Put the mask on your face and leave for 20 minutes, then wash it off with cool water. This mask is useful for dry skin inclined to irritation. It nourishes well, calming and rejuvenating skin.

✔ Cream-apricot mask

- 1 apricot

- Curds or sour cream

Mix the apricot pulp with the curds or sour cream in equal proportions (1 tablespoon of each ingredient).Put the mask on your face for 15-20 minutes, then wash it off with room temperature water.

✔ Peach mask 1

- 1 peach

- 1 teaspoon of lemon juice

Mash the peach pulp well, adding 1 teaspoon of lemon juice and apply to the face for 10-15 minutes. Then wash it off with warm water.

✔ Peach mask 2

- 1 tablespoon of peach juice

- Half a tablespoon of honey

- Half a tablespoon of fresh curds

Mix 1 tablespoon of peach juice with half a tablespoon of honey and half a tablespoon of fresh curds. Apply this mixture to your face for 10-15 minutes. Wash it off with soft cool water. This mask is useful for dry sensitive skin.

✔ Apple mask

- 1 apple

- 1 tablespoon of cream or sour cream

- 1 egg yolk

Grate the apple on a small plastic grater. Add 1 tablespoon of cream or sour cream and 1 egg yolk. Stir thoroughly and apply this mixture to your face. Leave the mask for 10-15 minutes. Wash it off with warm water. This mask nourishes and freshens skin. This vitamin mask can be created with the use of grated apples only, however, such an alternative requires greasing dry skin with vegetable oil beforehand.

✔ Orange mask

- 2 tablespoons of fresh fat curds

- Orange juice (1/2 of orange)

- 1 teaspoon of almond or nut oil

Carefully stir 2 tablespoons of fresh fat curds into the orange juice (1/2 of orange) and 1 teaspoon of almond or nut oil. Apply this mixture to your face and leave the mask for 15 minutes. Wash it off with warm water. This nourishing mask freshens and smoothes skin.

✔ Avocado mask

- Avocado

- 1 teaspoon of sesame, coconut or almond oil

Peel the avocado, remove seeds and mash it into pulp. Add 1 teaspoon of sesame, coconut or almond oil, stir and put the mask on the skin of your face and neck. Leave the mask for 20 minutes. Then remove it with a wet napkin.

✔ **Watermelon mask**

- 1 teaspoon of water-melon juice

- 1 egg yolk

- 1 teaspoon of vegetable oil

- Rye flour

Mix 1 teaspoon of watermelon juice with 1 egg yolk and 1 teaspoon of vegetable oil. Add rye flour to make it thicker. Apply this mixture to your face for 15-20 minutes, then wash it off with cool water or linden flowers tincture.

✔ **Melon mask**

- 2 tablespoons of melon pulp

- 1 egg yolk

- 1 tablespoon of almond or olive oil

Mix 2 tablespoons of melon pulp with the egg yolk and 1 tablespoon of almond or olive oil and put this mixture on your face. Leave the mask for 10-15 minutes. Wash it off with warm water.

✔ **Sea-buckthorn mask**

- Sea-buckthorn juice or berries

- 1 tablespoon of fresh sour cream

Mix 1 tablespoon of sea-buckthorn juice or kneaded berries with 1 tablespoon of fresh sour cream and apply this mixture to your face. Leave the mask for 10 minutes, then wash it off with warm water. Sea-buckthorn is especially useful for dry skin and is nourishing and softening.

✔ Strawberry mask

- Large ripe strawberries

- 1 tablespoon of olive oil

Mash some large ripe strawberries, mix with 1 tablespoon of olive oil and apply this mixture to your face. Leave the mask for 10 minutes and wash it off with warm water.

✔ Aloe and strawberry mask

- 2 teaspoons of dried tutsan herb

- 1 tablespoon of crushed aloe

- 2-3 strawberries

- Half a teaspoon of vegetable oil

Mix 2 teaspoons of dried tutsan herb with 1 tablespoon of crushed aloe. Mash 2-3 strawberries and add half a teaspoon of vegetable oil. Stir everything carefully and apply to your face with a cotton wool ball. In 15-20 minutes wash the mask off with warm water.

✔ Gooseberry mask

- Gooseberries

Apply ripe gooseberry juice and pulp to your face, leave for 20 minutes, then wash it off. This mask nourishes and bleaches dry skin.

✔ Raspberry mask

- Raspberries

- 1 egg yolk

Mix 1 tablespoon of ripe kneaded raspberries with a whipped egg yolk. Apply to your face for 20 minutes. Then wash it off with cool water. For sensitive skin add some sour cream or fat curds to the mixture. This mask is useful for dry skin inclined to the occurrence of wrinkles.

✔ Black currant mask

- Black currants
- 1 teaspoon of honey
- 1 teaspoon of sour cream

Add 1 teaspoon of honey and sour cream to 1 tablespoon of black currant pulp. Apply this mixture to your face for 15-20 minutes, then wash it off.

✔ Grape mask with almond oil

- 1 egg yolk
- 1 teaspoon of grape juice
- 1 teaspoon of sour cream
- 1 teaspoon of almond oil
- Rye flour

Knead the egg yolk, add 1 teaspoon of grape juice, sour cream and almond oil to it and stir, adding rye flour to the consistency of a thick cream. Put the mask on your face for 15-20 minutes, then wash it off with cool water.

✔ Dill mask

- 1 tablespoon of crushed dill greens
- 1 teaspoon of olive oil
- Oatmeal

Mix 1 tablespoon of crushed dill greens with 1 teaspoon of olive oil, add some oatmeal and stir to the consistency of gruel. Apply the mask to your face and leave for 10-15 minutes. Then wash it off with soft warm water.

✔ Tea mask

- 1 teaspoon of mayonnaise

- 1 teaspoon of nourishing cream

- 1 teaspoon of strong tea

- Milk

- Water

Mix 1 teaspoon of mayonnaise and 1 teaspoon of nourishing cream while adding 1 teaspoon of strong tea little-by-little. Wipe your face and neck with warm milk before applying this mask. Apply the first layer of the mask with light circular movements, then in 2-3 minutes apply the second layer. In 10-15 minutes remove the mask with a solution of milk with water (1:1).

Creams, oils and ointments for dry facial skin

✔ Cucumber cream

- 10 g of beeswax

- 40 ml of peach, almond or olive oil

- 2 tablespoons of cucumber juice

Melt 10g of beeswax on a water bath. Add 40 ml of peach, almond or olive oil and 2 tablespoons of cucumber juice, stir thoroughly. Let the cream cool down.

✔ Carrot cream

- 1 egg yolk

- 1 tablespoons of fresh carrot juice

- 20 g of beeswax

- 1 tablespoons of olive, sunflower or any other vegetable oil

Mix the egg yolk with 1 tablespoon of fresh carrot juice. Melt 20 g of beeswax on a water bath and mix with1 tablespoon of olive, sunflower or any other vegetable oil. Turn off the heat, add carrot mixture, stir carefully and let the cream cool down.

✔ **Peach cream**

- 10 g of lanolin

- 40 ml of peach oil

- 20 ml of distilled water

Melt 10 g of lanolin on a water bath, add 40 ml of peach oil and 20 ml of distilled water. Use this cream for the night.

✔ **Peach cream with cocoa oil**

- 40 ml of peach cream

- 25 g of lanolin

- 5 g of cocoa oil

- Lemon juice

- 20 ml of distilled water

Mix 40 ml of peach cream with 25 g of lanolin and 5 g of cocoa oil melted on a water bath. Add several drops of lemon juice and 20 ml of distilled water. Use as a night-time nourishing cream for dry skin.

✔ **Pear cream**

- 1 tablespoon of pear

- 25 ml of peach, apricot or almond oil

- 1 egg yolk

- 5 teaspoons of fresh cream

Mash 1 tablespoon of pear into pulp, add 25 ml of hot peach, apricot or almond oil, leave to infuse in a closed vessel for 3 days and filter. Whip 1 egg yolk with 5 teaspoons of fresh cream and add this mix to the oil and pear infusion. Store the prepared cream in a refrigerator.

✔ Strawberry cream

- 1 tablespoon of lanolin
- 1 tablespoon of oatmeal
- 100 ml of strawberry juice
- 5 drops of camphor spirit

Melt 1 tablespoon of lanolin on a water bath and add 1 tablespoon of oatmeal while stirring slowly. Remove the mixture from the water bath, add 100 ml of strawberry juice and 5 drops of camphor spirit. Let the cream cool down and store in a refrigerator for no longer than a week.

✔ Black currant cream

- 2 tablespoons of fresh butter
- 1 teaspoon of honey
- 1 teaspoon of olive or almond oil
- 2 tablespoons of black currants
- 2 teaspoons of camphor spirit

Melt 2 tablespoons of fresh butter on a water bath. Mix with 1 teaspoon of honey, 1 teaspoon of olive or almond oil and 2 tablespoons of black currants mashed into pulp. Stir thoroughly. Add 2 teaspoons of camphor spirit little-by-little and let it cool down.

✔ Ashberry cream

- 2 tablespoons of red ashberry pulp

- 1 tablespoon of peach, almond or olive oil

- 50 ml of whipped cream

Mix 2 tablespoons of red ashberry pulp with 1 tablespoon of peach, almond or olive oil and heat on a water bath for 30 minutes. Let it cool down, add 50 ml of whipped cream and stir carefully. Store the prepared cream in a refrigerator and apply it to your face for the night.

✓ **Rose cream**

- Rose petals (5 pink roses)

- 10 g of beeswax

- 50 g of fresh butter

- 1 teaspoon of vitamin A oil solution

Crush the rose petals carefully. Melt 10 g of beeswax on a water bath, add 50 g of fresh butter and rose petals, stir carefully and remove from the water bath. Then add 1 teaspoon of vitamin A oil solution, stir again and let the cream cool down.

✓ **Chamomile cream**

- 1 tablespoon of chamomile flowers

- 100 ml of boiling water

- 50 g of fresh butter

- 2 teaspoons of castor oil

- Half a teaspoon of glycerin

- 1 tablespoon of camphor spirit

Add 1 tablespoon of chamomile flowers to 100 ml of boiling water, let it infuse for two hours and filter. Add 50 g of fresh butter (melted on a water bath while stirring it slowly), 2 teaspoons of castor oil, half a teaspoon of glycerin, 2 tablespoons of chamomile tincture and 1 tablespoon of camphor spirit. Stir well and let it cool down. Use this cream for dry skin prone to inflammation. Apply this cream for 20-30 minutes, then remove the remains with a napkin.

✓ Birch cream

- Birch buds
- Nettle leaves
- 50 ml of boiling water
- 10 g of beeswax
- 50 g of fresh butter
- 1 tablespoon of olive, sesame or almond oil
- 2 teaspoons of vitamin A oil solution

Add half a tablespoon of birch buds and nettle leaf mixture to 50 ml of boiling water, leave to infuse in a closed vessel for 30 minutes and filter. Melt 10 g of beeswax on a water bath, add 50 g of fresh butter, 1 tablespoon of olive, sesame or almond oil, 2 teaspoons of vitamin A oil solution and 1 tablespoon of birch tincture. Stir until you get a consistent texture and let it cool down.

✓ Almond-rose oil

- 30 g of cocoa oil
- 60 ml of almond oil
- 3-4 drops of rose essential oil

Melt 30 g of cocoa oil on a water bath, remove from the heat and add 60 ml of almond oil. Let it cool down and add 3-4 drops of rose essential oil. Stir well and pour into a small bottle. Use this oil for cleansing the skin of your face. Apply the oil and remove it with a napkin or a cotton wool ball moistened in hot water for some minutes. Then rinse your face with cool water.

Skin care recipes for combined facial skin

Combined facial skin (p.126)

Lotions, herbal tinctures and cream for combined facial skin (p.127)

Masks for combined facial skin (p.129)

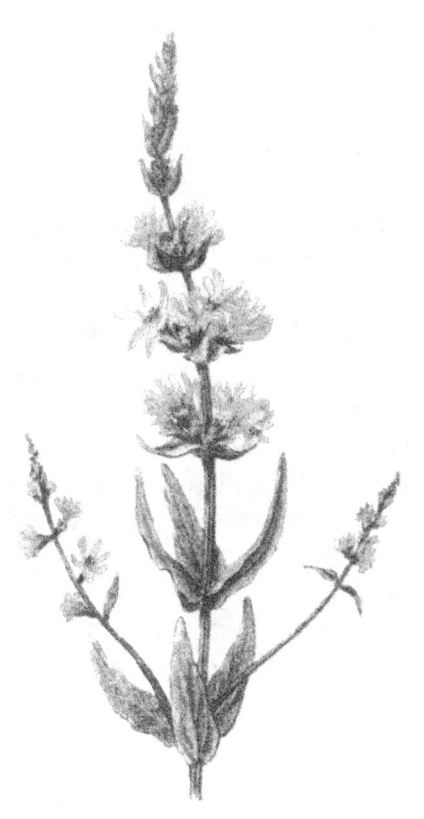

Combined facial skin

Combined skin occurs rather frequently. It is characterized by an uneven distribution of grease on different face areas. The skin is oily around the nose, forehead and chin (the so-called T-zone), constantly shiny and frequently becoming covered with acne or pimples. Around the eyes and cheeks the skin is gentle and dry, sometimes peeling and prone to wrinkles. It's vital to pay attention to your combined skin type and apply different products to different areas. Combined skin usually turns into normal skin with age.

Combined facial skin reacts badly to water and soap. Therefore it is recommended that you cleanse the face and neck with herbal extracts (calendula, mint, sage) in the morning and use cleansing creams, chamomile tincture or tea with milk in the evening. First wipe your skin two to three times with cotton wool balls moistened in full cream milk, and then moisten your face with a large amount of tea with milk, mixed in a 1:1 proportion. After washing the face, dry it with a piece of cotton wool, wipe your nose and chin with a lotion and apply nourishing cream. Another possible action is as follows: apply cream and masks for oily skin to oily areas of your face, and cream and masks for dry skin to dry areas. Apply cream to your skin each time after washing, and apply masks once a week.

Lotions, herbal tinctures and cream for combined facial skin

✔ Watermelon-peach lotion

- Watermelon juice

- Peach juice

Mix watermelon and peach juices in equal parts and wipe the dry areas of your face. Watermelon clears skin well while the peach moistens and nourishes it.

✔ Dandelion lotion

- 1 glass of crushed dandelion with roots

- 200 ml of vodka

- Water

Add 1 glass of crushed fresh dandelion with roots to 200 ml of vodka in a glass jar, seal it tightly and leave to infuse for 10 days in a dark place. Then filter, dilute with water (1:2) and wipe oily areas of your face with this lotion 2-3 times a day.

✔ Mint lotion

- Half a tablespoon of peppermint leaves

- 100 ml of water

- 100 ml of unfiltered beer

Add half a tablespoon of peppermint leaves to 100 ml of water, heat on a water bath for 15 minutes, let it infuse for 45 minutes and filter. Add 100 ml of unfiltered beer to this infusion and use as a lotion for the dry areas of combined skin.

✔ Chamomile tincture

- 3 tablespoons of chamomile flowers

- 200 ml of water

Add 3 tablespoons of chamomile flowers to 200 ml of water, heat on a water bath for 15 minutes, leave to infuse at room temperature for 45 minutes and wipe the oily areas of your skin with the extract.

✔ Grapefruit peel cosmetic water for facial cleansing

- Grapefruit peel

- Water

You can prepare cosmetic water for cleansing your face with the use of a grapefruit peel: place the peel into a glass jar and fill with cold water. Filter the water after one day. Rinse your face with this water in the morning and in the evening or wipe with a cotton wool ball moistened in it.

✔ Vitamin cream for combined facial skin

- Lemon peel (2 lemons)

- 100 g of margarine

- 3 tablespoons of vegetable oil

- 1 egg yolk

- 1 teaspoon of honey

- Lemon juice (1 lemon)

- 10 drops of vitamin A oil solution

- 1 tablespoon of mayonnaise

- 1 tablespoon of camphor spirit

Make a tincture out of 2 lemons peel. Blend 100 g of margarine with 3 tablespoons of vegetable oil, 1 yolk and 1 teaspoon of honey. Add lemon juice little-by-little, 10 drops of vitamin A oil solution and 1 tablespoon of mayonnaise,1 tablespoon of camphor spirit and lemon peel tincture.

Masks for combined facial skin

✔ **Yeast mask**

- 1 tablespoon of yeast

- Water

- 1 tablespoon of kefir, yoghurt or curdled milk

- 1 teaspoon of baking soda

Break 1 tablespoon of yeast in a small amount of warm water, add 1 tablespoon of kefir, yoghurt or curdled milk and 1 teaspoon of baking soda. Stir well and apply the mask to oily skin zones. Leave for 15 minutes, then wash it off with warm water. This mask clears pores well and removes inflammations.

✔ **Cleansing peach mask**

- Half a peach

- 1 tablespoon of cognac

Mash and rub the pulp of half a peach through a sieve, then mix it with 1 tablespoon of cognac. Apply to your face for 10-15 minutes, then wash it off with warm water.

✔ **Cleansing carrot and turnip mask**

- 1 carrot

- 1 turnip

Boil a carrot and turnip, then mash them until you get a consistent texture. Apply to your skin for 10-15 minutes.

✔ **Kefir mask**

- 1 tablespoon of low-fat kefir

- 1 tablespoon of oatmeal

Mix 1 tablespoon of low-fat kefir with 1 tablespoon of oatmeal and put this mixture on the skin of your face. Leave the mask for 15 minutes, then wash it off with warm water and apply a nourishing cream. This mask moistens combined skin well.

✓ Egg-lemon mask

- 1 egg white

- Half a teaspoon of lemon juice

Whip the egg white and add half a teaspoon of lemon juice. Apply this mixture to oily zones of your skin and leave the mask for 20 minutes. Wash it off with warm, then with cool water.

✓ Almond mask

- 3-4 peeled almonds

- 100 ml of water

- Half a small cucumber

- 2 teaspoons of oat flakes

- 1 teaspoon of blue clay

Add 3-4 peeled almonds to 100 ml of water and crush in a blender. Grate half a small cucumber on a small plastic grater, wring juice out, add the cucumber paste to the almond mixture and stir. Then add 2 teaspoons of oat flakes and 1 teaspoon of blue clay. Stir carefully and apply the mixture to your face, massaging it slightly. Leave the mask for 15 minutes, then wash it off with warm water.

✓ Cucumber mask

- 1 small cucumber

- 1 egg white

- 70 ml of unfiltered beer

Peel 1 small cucumber and grate it on a small plastic grater, mix with 1 whipped egg white. Add 70 ml of unfiltered beer and put this mixture on your face. Cover the mask with a gauze napkin. Leave it for 15 minutes, then wash it off with cool water.

✔ Vegetable mask with lemon

- 1 tablespoon of carrot juice
- 1 tablespoon of cucumber juice
- 1 tablespoon of lemon juice
- 1 tablespoon of starch

Mix 1 tablespoon of carrot, cucumber and lemon juices with 1 tablespoon of starch and apply this mixture to the skin of your face with a cotton wool ball. Leave it for 15-20 minutes, then wash it off with warm water. This mask vitaminizes, softens and freshens skin.

✔ Yolk mask

- 1 egg yolk
- 1 teaspoon of cream

Mix 1 whipped egg yolk with 1 teaspoon of cream and apply this mixture to the dry zones of your skin. Leave the mask for 20 minutes, then wash it off with warm water and rinse the face with cool water.

✔ Sour-cream-carrot mask

- 2 tablespoons of sour cream
- 1 egg yolk
- 1 teaspoon of carrot juice

Whip 2 tablespoons of sour cream with the egg yolk, add 1 teaspoon of carrot juice and mix well. Apply this mask to dry areas of your skin and leave for 15-20 minutes. Wash it off with warm water.

✔ Curd mask

- 2 teaspoons of curds
- 2 teaspoons of wheat sprout oil
- 1 teaspoon of parsley juice

Mix 2 teaspoons of curds with 2 teaspoons of wheat sprout oil and add 1 teaspoon of parsley juice. Apply this paste to dry zones of your skin, leave for 15 minutes, wash it off with cool water or herbal tincture (mint, nettle, oregano) and apply a nourishing cream.

✔ Honey mask

- 1 egg yolk
- 1 tablespoon of honey
- 1 tablespoon of almond or nut oil
- Linden or mint tincture

Mix the egg yolk with 1 tablespoon of honey, add 1 tablespoon of almond or nut oil and stir well. Put the mask on your face for 15-20 minutes, then wash it off with linden or mint tincture. This mask is useful for dry skin zones.

✔ Apple mask

- 1 apple
- 1 egg yolk
- 1 teaspoon of olive oil

Peel the apple and grate on a small plastic grater, mix it carefully with the egg yolk and 1 teaspoon of olive oil. Apply the mask to your face for 20 minutes, then wash it off with warm water.

This nourishing mask is suitable for combined skin (normal or dry).

✓ **Tonic mask with elder tincture**

- 200 ml of milk
- 2 tablespoons of oat flakes
- 2 tablespoons of elder tincture

Combine 200 ml of milk, 2 tablespoons of oat flakes and boil. When the mixture thickens, add the elder tincture. Apply a thick layer of this warm paste to your face and neck. Wash it off with warm water, and then rinse the face with cool water. This mask softens and tones skin.

✓ **Berry juice mask**

- 200 ml of fresh or frozen strawberry or currant juice
- 1 teaspoon of lanolin
- 1 teaspoon of oat flakes powder

First dissolve 1 teaspoon of lanolin on a water bath, and then add 1 teaspoon of oat flakes powder. Mix until you get a consistent texture and while continuing to mix, add 200 ml of berry juice little-by-little.

✓ **Aloe mask with marrow squash**

- Half a marrow squash
- 100 ml of kefir
- 1 tablespoon of crushed aloe
- 30 ml of tutsan tincture

Mince half a marrow and add 100 ml of kefir, 1 tablespoon of aloe and 30 ml of tutsan tincture; mix the ingredients carefully. Put the mask on your face for 20 minutes, then wash it off with cool water.

✓ Aloe and pumpkin mask

- 1 tablespoon of aloe

- 2 tablespoons of boiled pumpkin

- 2 tablespoons of a concentrated tutsan tincture (40 g of herb per 200 ml of water)

- 1 tablespoon of yarrow extract (30 g of herb per 200 ml of water)

Mix 1 tablespoon of aloe, 2 tablespoons of boiled pumpkin, 2 tablespoons of a concentrated tutsan tincture and 1 tablespoon of yarrow extract. Blend the ingredients until smooth and put a thin layer of this mixture on your face. After 10-15 minutes wash it off with warm water.

✓ Oat flake mask

- 2 tablespoons of oat flakes

- 1 egg white

- 1 tablespoon of rose water

Blend 2 tablespoons of oat flakes, 1 whipped egg white and 1 tablespoon of rose water (add a handful of rose petals to 250 ml of boiling water and let it infuse in a closed vessel for 30 minutes, then filter; keep rose water in glassware in a cool place). Stir carefully, put the resulting mask on your face and wash it off in 15-20 minutes.

✓ Mask with rosehips and lemon juice

- 2 teaspoons of crushed rosehips

- 2 teaspoons of sage leaves

- 1 teaspoon of peppermint

- 300 ml of boiling water

- Lemon juice (1/2 of lemon)

- Strong tea

Add 2 teaspoons of crushed rosehips, 2 teaspoons of sage leaves and 1 teaspoon of peppermint to 300 ml of boiling water and place on a water bath, covered, for 30 minutes. Cool this tincture a little and mix with the lemon juice; do not filter. Spread the thick herbal mask on a gauze napkin and then apply it to your face. Cover it with a thick double towel and after 15-20 minutes remove the remains of the mask by washing it off with warm strong tea. Let your skin dry by itself and apply moisturizing cream.

✓ Curd-honey-grape mask

- 1 teaspoon of curds
- 1 teaspoon of liquid honey
- 2 teaspoons of grape juice

Blend 1 teaspoon of curds with the same quantity of liquid honey and add 2 teaspoons of grape juice. Apply a thick layer of this mixture to your face and after 10-15 minutes wash it off with cold water.

Skin care recipes for withering facial skin

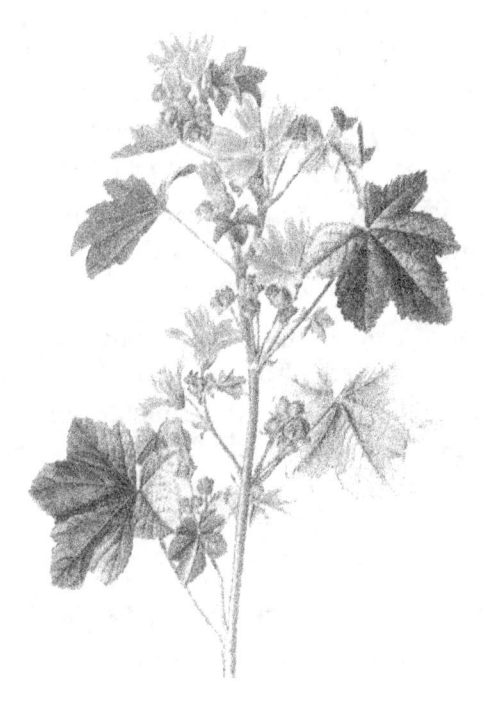

Withering skin

In the case of withering skin first signs can appear at the age of 35; main attention should be paid to the usage of nourishing and moisturizing products for stimulating skin metabolism.

In the morning, right after awakening, wipe the skin on your face, hands and neck with cosmetic milk and put cream, sour cream or kefir on it for 15-20 minutes.

Wash off the mask with a strong water jet at a pleasant temperature after 20 minutes. Then wipe the skin on your face, neck and chest skin with an ice cube with fast circular movements. It is better to begin with a single wiping, gradually increasing it to 5-7 times. At the end apply some cream. In 15 minutes remove the surplus of cream with a paper napkin.

For evening cleaning of withering skin use chamomile, mint, tutsan, sage or linden flower tinctures as well as orange or lemon juices dissolved half-and-half with water.

After washing apply a nourishing cream on damp skin using cotton wool balls moistened in salted water, herbal tinctures, berry, fruit or vegetable juice. In 30-40 minutes remove the surplus of cream with a paper napkin. Use cream after wash and apply masks 2-3 times a week.

Herbal tinctures, decoctions and infusions for withering facial skin care

✔ **Rosemary tincture**

- 1 tablespoon of crushed rosemary leaves

- 200 ml of dry red wine or vodka

Add 1 tablespoon of crushed rosemary leaves to 200 ml of dry red wine (for dry and normal skin) or vodka (for oily skin), leave to infuse for 6 weeks, stirring periodically, then filter and wipe your face and neck with this tincture twice a day. This tincture smoothes wrinkles, making skin elastic. Keep it in a cool place.

✔ Rose tincture

- Fresh rose petals
- Vodka

Fill a half liter bottle with fresh rose petals and pour vodka over them to the brim. Leave to infuse in a dark place for a month. Then filter the tincture and wipe your face with it. This tincture rejuvenates skin, making it elastic.

✔ Aloe infusion

- 50 g of biostimulating aloe leaves
- Half a liter of cold water

Crush 50 g of biostimulating aloe leaves, add half a liter of cold water and leave to infuse for 2 hours. Then bring this infusion to a boil on a low heat, let it cool down, filter and use for wiping withering skin on your face and neck. This effective remedy prevents aging of skin and the formation of wrinkles. Keep this infusion in a refrigerator.

✔ Melissa infusion

- 1 tablespoon of melissa leaves
- 200 ml of boiled water

Wipe withering skin with melissa infusion instead of washing. The infusion is prepared: 1 tablespoon of leaves per 200 ml of boiled water.

✔ Rosemary infusion

- Rosemary leaves and flowers

- 200 ml of boiling water

Add rosemary leaves and flowers to 200 ml of boiling water in a thermos, let it infuse for 30-45 minutes and filter. Wipe or wash your face with the infusion. After washing do not wipe it dry. Consistent application of rosemary infusion for lengthy periods of time keeps skin young, preventing the occurrence of wrinkles.

✓ **Linden flowers and raspberry leaf infusion**

- 1 tablespoon of crushed raspberry leaves

- 1 tablespoon of linden flowers

- 200 ml of water

Add 1 tablespoon of crushed raspberry leaves and 1 tablespoon of linden flowers to 200 ml of water, heat on a water bath for 15 minutes and let it infuse for 45 minutes. Then filter and wipe your face with the infusion. This is an effective remedy for loose skin and wrinkles.

✓ **Oak bark and linden infusion**

- 1 teaspoon of crushed oak bark

- 1 tablespoon of linden flowers

- 300-400 ml of boiled water

Mix 1 teaspoon of crushed oak bark with 1 tablespoon of linden flowers. And add 300-400 ml of boiled water, leave to infuse for 2 hours, then filter. Wipe loose, flabby, wrinkle-prone skin with this infusion in the morning and in the evening instead of washing.

✓ **Anise infusion**

- 1 teaspoon of anise fruits

- 100 ml of water

Knead 1 teaspoon of anise fruits, add 100 ml of water, cover and heat on a water bath. Let it infuse for 45 minutes and then filter. Wipe your face with the infusion. It rejuvenates dry wrinkled skin, slightly bleaching it and eliminating edemas.

✔ Rose petal infusion

- 2 tablespoons of crushed rose petals
- 200 ml of boiling water

Use rose petal infusion for wiping dry withering skin. To prepare the infusion add 2 tablespoons of crushed petals to 200 ml of boiled water and let it infuse in a closed vessel at room temperature until it cools down.

✔ Plantain extract

- 2 tablespoons of crushed plantain leaves
- 200 ml of water

Add 2 tablespoons of crushed plantain leaves to 200 ml of water, heat on a water bath for 30 minutes, let it cool down in a closed vessel at room temperature and filter. Freeze this infusion in moulds and wipe oily wrinkled skin with the resulting ice cubes.

✔ Peppermint infusion

- 1 tablespoon of crushed peppermint leaves
- 200 ml of boiling water

Add 1 tablespoon of crushed peppermint leaves to 200 ml of boiling water, let it infuse in a warm place for 30 minutes and filter. Freeze the infusion in moulds and wipe oily wrinkled skin with the resulting ice cubes. This infusion freshens and tones skin, smoothing out wrinkles.

✔ Parsley extract

- 25 g of parsley greens

- 250 ml of water

Add 25 g of parsley greens to 250 ml of water, boil for 15 minutes, let it cool down and filter. Freeze the extract in moulds and wipe your face with the resulting ice cubes. This extract tones skin and prevents wrinkles.

✓ **Cucumber water**

- 40 ml of cucumber juice

- 40 ml of tutsan extract

- 20 ml of rose or distilled water

Mix 40 ml of cucumber juice, 40 ml of tutsan extract (add half a tablespoon of tutsan herb to 200 ml of water, heat on a water bath for 30 minutes and filter) and 20 ml of rose water or distilled water. Wipe the skin of your face to refresh and smooth it out.

Lotions for withering facial skin

✓ **Rejuvenating lotion**

- 50 ml of biostimulating aloe juice

- 50 ml of kalanchoe juice

- 25 ml of plantain juice

- 25 ml of Rhaponticum carthamoides tincture

- 30 ml of distilled water

- 15 ml of glycerin

Mix 50 ml of biostimulating aloe juice, 50 ml of kalanchoe juice, 25 ml of fresh plantain juice and 25 ml of Rhaponticum carthamoides tincture. Add 30 ml of distilled water and 15 ml of glycerin. Wipe your face 2-3 times a week for 1-2 months with this lotion. Shake the lotion before application.

✔ Quince lotion

- 1 egg white
- 70 ml of quince juice
- 30 ml of camphor spirit

Mix the egg white whipped into froth with 70 ml of quince juice and 30 ml of camphor spirit. Wipe porous withering skin with the lotion. It freshens, smoothes and bleaches skin.

✔ Lemon-flower lotion

- 2 tablespoons of white lily petals
- 2 tablespoons of rose petals
- 2 tablespoons of jasmine petals
- Water
- Dried lemon peel (2 lemons)
- Lemon juice (2 lemons)
- 2 teaspoon of honey
- 1 teaspoon of olive oil
- 1 tablespoon of cream
- 20 ml of cologne

Prepare white lily, rose and jasmine petals infusions separately (add 3 tablespoons of petals to 200 ml of water and heat on a water bath for 15 minutes). Add grated dried lemon peel to 100 ml of boiled water and let it infuse for 8-10 hours. Then filter, add lemon juice, 2 teaspoons of honey, 1 teaspoon of olive oil, 1 tablespoon of cream, 50 ml flower petal infusion, 20 ml of cologne and stir thoroughly. This lotion is perfect for withering flabby skin. Store it in a refrigerator.

✔ Flower lotion with avocado

- 2 ripe avocados

- White lilies petals (2 white lilies)
- Pink roses petals (4 pink roses)
- Half a liter of vodka
- 50 ml of distilled water
- Half a tablespoon of glycerin
- Lemon juice

Knead two ripe avocados and add the lower petals. Add this mix to half a liter of vodka. Leave to infuse for three weeks, then filter. Keep the tincture in a refrigerator and use for preparing lotion: add 50 ml of distilled water, half a tablespoon of glycerin and lemon juice to 50 ml of tincture. This lotion smoothes wrinkled skin.

✔ **Lotion with herbs**

- 10 g of peppermint leaves
- 10 g of rosemary leaves
- 10 g of calendula flowers
- 15 g of chamomile flowers
- Half a liter of dry white wine
- Vegetable oil

Add 10 g of peppermint leaves, 10 g of rosemary leaves, 10 g of calendula flowers and 15 g of chamomile flowers to half a liter of dry white wine, leave to infuse for 2 weeks and filter. In the case of early wrinkles wipe your face with this lotion every evening and then grease it with vegetable oil. This lotion makes skin healthy, refreshing it thoroughly.

✔ **Dill lotion**

- Dill greens
- 1 tablespoon of linden flowers
- 1 teaspoon of sage leaves

- 300 ml of boiling water

- 1 tablespoon of crushed greens of fennel

Add 1 tablespoon of linden flowers and 1 teaspoon of sage leaves to 300 ml of boiling water, leave to infuse for 2 hours and filter. Use this lotion for flabby wrinkled skin. Store it in a refrigerator.

✓ Plantain lotion

- Common plantain juice or infusion

- Fresh milk

Mix common plantain juice or infusion with fresh milk at a 1:1 ratio and use the lotion for cleansing withering wrinkled skin.

Rejuvenating masks for withering facial skin

✓ Aloe mask 1

- 1 aloe leaf

Crush 1 aloe leaf and put on your face for 10-15 minutes. Then wash it off first with warm, then with cool water. This mask tones skin and smoothes wrinkles.

✓ Aloe mask 2

- 1 teaspoon of aloe juice

- 1 teaspoon of olive oil

Mix 1 teaspoon of aloe juice and olive oil and put on your face for 10-15 minutes. Wash it off first with warm, then with cool water. The mask rejuvenates skin, preventing the occurrence of wrinkles.

✓ Aloe mask 3

- 1 egg yolk

- 1 teaspoon of aloe juice

- 1 tablespoon of sour cream

Mix the egg yolk with 1 teaspoon of aloe juice and 1 tablespoon of sour cream. Put this mixture on your face and neck in layers, each following layer should be applied when the previous one has dried. Procedure duration: 20-30 minutes. Wash the mask off with warm water and then rinse with cold.

✔ Mask with wheat bran

- 2 tablespoons of wheat bran

- 1 teaspoons of honey

- 2 tablespoons of tea mushroom tincture

Mix 2 tablespoons of wheat bran with 1 teaspoon of honey and 2 tablespoon of tea mushroom tincture. Apply the mask to the preliminarily cleared skin of your face and leave for 30 minutes, then wash it off with warm water. This mask is useful for dry withering skin.

✔ Blue clay mask 1

- 1 tablespoon of blue clay

- 1 tablespoon of whey or low-fat kefir

Mix 1 tablespoon of blue clay in 1 tablespoon of whey or low-fat kefir. Put the mask on your face, leave for 20 minutes (until it dries), then wash it off with cool water. This mask softens and tones skin, smoothing small wrinkles. It is enough to apply it once a week.

✔ Blue clay mask 2

- 1 tablespoon of lavender flowers

- 1 tablespoon of chamomile flowers

- 1 tablespoon of linden flowers

- 1 tablespoon of sage leaves

- Boiling water

- Blue clay

Add 1 tablespoon of each ingredient (lavender flowers, chamomile flowers, linden flowers and sage leaves) to some boiling water and stir to the consistency of liquid gruel. Leave to infuse for 10 minutes, let it cool down and mix with blue clay to a creamy consistency. Cool one part of this mixture in a refrigerator, warm the other on a water bath and spread gauze napkins with both mixtures. Then apply the warm mask first followed by the cold one to your face. Leave the mask for 5 minutes. Protect your eyes with cotton wool balls moistened in linden flower or calendula tincture. Carry out this procedure once a week. It is recommended for wrinkled skin.

✔ Blue clay mask 3

- 1 tablespoon of blue clay

- 1 tablespoon of cold milk

- 1 teaspoon of honey

Mix 1 tablespoon of blue clay in 1 tablespoon of cold milk and add 1 teaspoon of honey. Apply the mask for 20 minutes. Then wash it off with warm water. It tones tired loose skin.

✔ Yolk mask with beer

- 1 egg yolk

- Beer

Whisk the egg yolk with the beer and put this mixture on your face for 20 minutes. Then wash it off with cool water. It is recommended to apply this mask once a week.

✔ Potato mask with beer

- 1 raw potato

- 2 tablespoons of beer

- 1 egg yolk

Grate 1 raw potato on a small plastic grater, add 2 tablespoons of beer and 1 egg yolk. Stir well and apply this mixture to your face. Leave the mask for 10-15 minutes, then wash it off with cool water. Masks with beer smooth wrinkles well.

✔ Mustard mask

- 1 teaspoon of mustard powder

- 1 teaspoon of water

- 2 teaspoons of olive or sunflower-seed oil

Dissolve 1 teaspoon of mustard powder in1 teaspoon of water and mix with 2 teaspoons of olive or sunflower-seed oil. Apply this mixture to your face for 20 minutes. Wash it off with warm, then with cool water. This mask tones pale withering skin very well. However it is not recommended for use in the case of widened vessels and hypertrichosis.

✔ Rice flour mask

- 1 teaspoon of rice flour

- 1 teaspoon of sour cream

- 1 egg yolk

Mix 1 teaspoon of rice flour with 2 teaspoons of sour cream and 1 egg yolk. Apply this mixture to your face for 20 minutes. Then wash it off with warm water and rinse the face with cool.

✔ Linseed mask

- 1 tablespoon of linden flowers

- 250 ml of water

- 1 tablespoon of linseed flour

- 1 tablespoon of honey

- 10 ml of oil solution of vitamins A and E

To prepare the infusion add 1 tablespoon of linden flowers to 250 ml of water, heat on a water bath for 15 minutes, leave to infuse for 45 minutes and filter. Mix 1 tablespoon of linseed flour with 1 tablespoon of honey and 2 tablespoons of the linden flowers tincture. Add 10 ml of the oil solution of vitamins A and E. Apply this mixture to your face and leave for 15-20 minutes. Wash it off with warm water, then with cold water. This mask is recommended for withering facial skin.

✔ Oatmeal mask with sauerkraut juice

- 2 tablespoons of oatmeal

- 2 tablespoons of sauerkraut juice

Mix 2 tablespoons of oatmeal with 2 tablespoons of sauerkraut juice. Apply this mixture to your face for 20 minutes, then wash it off. This mask is recommended for loose wrinkled skin.

✔ Oatmeal mask with kefir

- 2 tablespoons of oatmeal

- Kefir or natural yoghurt

- Whey

Mix 2 tablespoons of oatmeal with the kefir or natural yoghurt to the consistency of sour cream. Apply this mixture to your face for 15-20 minutes, then wash it off with whey. This mask nourishes, softens and tones loose skin.

✔ Creamy-oatmeal mask

- 1 tablespoon of cream

- 1 tablespoon of oatmeal

- Pinch of salt

- Water

Mix 1 tablespoon of cream with 1 tablespoon of oatmeal. Add a pinch of salt and some water until you get a gruel consistency. Apply this mixture to your face for 15-20 minutes, then wash it off with warm water. This mask smoothes wrinkles and is useful for dry sensitive skin.

✔ **Oat flakes mask with herbs**

- Oat flakes

- Crushed yarrow herb

- Tutsan herb

- Oregano herb

- Boiling water

Mince the oat flakes in a mincing machine and then mix with 1 tablespoon of crushed yarrow, tutsan and oregano herbs, taken in equal proportions. Add some boiling water and stir to the consistency of thick gruel. Put the mask on your face, leave for 20 minutes, then wash it off with cool some water. This mask calms and rejuvenates skin and smoothes small wrinkles.

✔ **Yolk mask with oatmeal**

- 1 egg yolk

- 1 teaspoon of oatmeal

- Half a teaspoon of honey

- Half a teaspoon of lemon juice

- Half a teaspoon of olive or almond oil

Knead the egg yolk with 1 teaspoon of honey. Add half a teaspoon of lemon juice and half a teaspoon of olive or almond oil. Mix it well with 1 teaspoon of oatmeal. Apply this mixture to your face for 15-20 minutes. Then wash it off with cool water. This mask clears, nourishes and tones a withering skin that peels.

✔ Rye flour mask with egg yolk

- 1 tablespoon of rye flour
- Warm milk
- 1 egg yolk

Dissolve 1 tablespoon of rye flour in warm milk to the consistency of thick sour cream and mix with the egg yolk. Apply this mixture to your face, leave for 15 minutes and wash it off with warm water. This mask smoothes wrinkles.

✔ Almond bran mask with herbs

- 1 teaspoon of rosemary leaves
- 1 teaspoon of tarragon leaves
- 1 teaspoon of parsley greens
- 100 ml of hot milk
- 2 tablespoons of almond bran

Add 1 teaspoon of rosemary leaves, tarragon leaves and parsley greens to 100 ml of hot milk, let it infuse, filter and add 2 tablespoons of almond bran to the herbal infusion. Stir well. Apply the mask to your face and leave for 10-15 minutes. Wash it off with cool water. This mask clears and tones withering skin, smoothes wrinkles.

✔ Yeast mask 1

- 20 g of yeast
- Warm milk
- 1 teaspoon of peach or apple juice
- 1 egg yolk

Break 20 g of yeast in the warm milk, add 1 teaspoon of peach or apple juice and the egg yolk, blend thoroughly and put this mixture on your face. Leave the mask for 10-15 minutes. Then wash it off with warm, then with cold water. It tones and nourishes wrinkled withering skin well.

✔ Yeast mask 2

- 20 g of yeast

- Red ashberry juice

- 1 egg white

Break 20 g of yeast in the red ashberry juice and add 1 egg white. Leave the mask for 20 minutes. Wash it off with warm, then with cold water.

✔ Honey-milk mask

- 1 tablespoon of honey

- 1 tablespoon of milk

Mix 1 tablespoon of honey with 1 tablespoon of milk and apply to your face with a cotton wool ball for 10-15 minutes. Then wash it off with warm water. This mask is useful for pale withering skin. It is not recommended in the case of widened vessels.

✔ Honey mask with linden flowers

- 1 tablespoon of linden flowers

- 250 ml of water

- 1 teaspoon of honey

Add 1 tablespoon of linden flowers to 250 ml of water, heat on a water bath for15 minutes, leave to infuse for 45 minutes and filter. Add 1 teaspoon of honey to this infusion, moisten a gauze napkin and apply to your face for 15-20 minutes. Wash it off with warm, then with cold water and spread your face with a nourishing cream. This mask rejuvenates skin effectively.

✔ Curds-salt mask

- 1 tablespoon of fresh curds
- 2 tablespoons of sour cream
- Half a teaspoon of table salt
- Cold milk

Blend 1 tablespoon of fresh curds with 2 tablespoons of sour cream, add half a teaspoon of table salt and knead it thoroughly. Put this mask on your face for 15-20 minutes, then wash it off with a cotton wool ball moistened in cold milk.. This mask tones and softens dry withering skin.

✔ Curds-carrot mask

- 2 tablespoons of curds
- 1 tablespoon of fresh carrot juice

Blend 2 tablespoons of curds with 1 tablespoon of fresh carrot juice and put this mixture on the skin of your face and neck. Leave the mask for 10-15 minutes. Wash it off with warm, then with cold water. This mask tones and nourishes withering skin.

✔ Curds-lemon mask

- 1 tablespoon of curds
- 5-10 drops of lemon juice or a lemon slice

Mix 1 tablespoon of curds with 5-10 drops of lemon juice or with a crushed lemon slice. Put this mask on your face and leave for 20-30 minutes. It moistens skin well and smoothes wrinkles. If your skin is very dry, you can grease it with warmed olive oil.

✔ Curds-sour cream mask with ashberry

- 2 tablespoon of curds
- 1 tablespoon of sour cream

- 1 egg yolk

- 1 teaspoon of honey

- Red ashberries

Blend 2 tablespoons of curds with 1 tablespoon of sour cream, add the egg yolk, 1 teaspoon of honey and 1 teaspoon of finely mashed red ashberries. Stir thoroughly and apply the mask to your face. Leave for 20-30 minutes. Then wash it off with warm water and rinse your face with cool water. This rejuvenating mask is useful for withering skin.

✔ Curds-honey mask with herbs

- Rosemary leaves

- Hop cones

- Linden flowers

- Chamomile flowers

- 1 tablespoon of curds

- 1 tablespoon of honey

- 1 cube of mint ice

Mince rosemary leaves, hop cones, linden flowers and chamomile flowers taken in equal parts. And add water so that it covers the mixture and boil. Let it infuse for 10 minutes and mix 1 tablespoon of herbs with 1 tablespoon of curds and 1 tablespoon of honey. Apply the mask to your face, leave for 20-30 minutes. Then wash it off with warm water and wipe your face with a cube of mint ice. This mask narrows pores, calms tired skin and is useful when skin is showing signs of withering.

✔ Cucumber mask 1

- 1 cucumber

- 1 teaspoon of honey

Grate 1 fresh cucumber on a small plastic grater, add 1 teaspoon of honey and apply this mixture to your face. Leave the mask for

10-15 minutes. Then wash it off with warm water, or with rose petals infusion. This mask is recommended for withering skin.

✔ Cucumber mask 2

- Overripe cucumbers

Grate overripe cucumbers on a small plastic grater and apply the pulp to your face. Leave the mask for 10-15 minutes. It helps to smooth wrinkles.

✔ Cucumber mask 3

- 2 tablespoons of cucumber juice

- 1 tablespoon of cream

- Rose water

Mix 2 tablespoons of cucumber juice with 2 tablespoons of cream and apply this mixture to your face. Leave the mask for 20-25 minutes then wash it off with rose water. Cucumber masks are useful for withering skin with enlarged/widened pores. They make it healthier, smooth and bleach skin. Another option is putting cucumber slices, cucumber peel or grated cucumber pulp on the face. Procedures are carried out before sleep 2-3 times a week within a month.

✔ Melon mask

- 2 tablespoons of ripe melon pulp

- Half a tablespoon of grape or lemon juice

- 1 teaspoon of starch (potato, rice or corn)

Mix 2 tablespoons of the melon pulp with half a tablespoon of grape or lemon juice and 1 teaspoon of starch. Put this mask on your face, leave for 20 minutes, then wash it off with warm water. The mask is useful for withering facial skin.

✓ Pea mask 1

- 2 tablespoons of green peas flour

- Whey

Mix 2 tablespoons of green peas flour with whey to the consistency of gruel. Apply this mixture to the face and leave for 10-15 minutes. Remove with a dry cotton wool ball and rinse your face with warm, then with cool water. This mask clears and rejuvenates skin, makes it matte and elastic, smoothes wrinkles. It is suitable for any type of skin, but it is more useful for oily skin.

✓ Pea mask 2

- Boiled green peas, kneaded

- 1 egg yolk

- 2 tablespoons of fresh apple juice

Mix 2 tablespoons of kneaded boiled green peas with the egg yolk and 2 tablespoons of fresh apple juice. Apply this mixture to your face, leave for 20 minutes, then wash it off with warm water. This mask nourishes and smoothes dry wrinkled skin well. It can be used every other day within a month.

✓ Haricot mask

- Boiled haricot, kneaded

- 1 teaspoon of lemon juice

- Olive oil

Mix 2 tablespoons of kneaded boiled haricot with 1 teaspoon of lemon juice and add the olive oil. Stir to the consistency of thick sour cream. Apply this warm mixture to your face, leave the mask for 20 minutes, wash it off with warm, then with cool water. This mask calms, nourishes and softens dry withering skin, smoothes small wrinkles.

✔ Sweet pepper mask

- 1 sweet pepper
- 1 teaspoon of milk
- 1 teaspoon of honey
- 1 tablespoon of oatmeal

Grate 1 sweet pepper on a small plastic grater, add 1 teaspoon of milk and honey, 1 tablespoon of oatmeal and stir carefully. Apply this mixture to your face for 15-20 minutes and wash it off with warm water. This mask rejuvenates and freshens skin.

✔ Mask with avocado and tea mushroom infusion

- Avocado
- 1 egg yolk
- 2 tablespoons of tea mushroom infusion
- 1 tablespoon of wheat sprouts oil
- Half a teaspoon of lemon juice

Whip the egg yolk, adding 2 tablespoons of tea mushroom infusion little-by-little and1 tablespoon of wheat sprouts oil. Then add 1 teaspoon of kneaded pulp of avocado and half a teaspoon of lemon juice. Stir well and put this mixture on your face. Leave the mask for an hour, then wash it off with cool water. This mask is useful for dry withering skin.

✔ Topinambour mask

- Topinambour
- 1 egg yolk or 1 tablespoon of sour cream

Mix 1 tablespoon of the tuber of topinambour, peeled and grated on a small grater, with 1 egg yolk or 1 tablespoon of fresh sour cream and apply this mixture to your face. Leave for 20-30 minutes. Then wash it off with warm water. It is necessary to apply this mask twice a week in the case of flabby wrinkled skin.

✔ Carrot cream mask

- 1 small carrot
- 1 tablespoon of cream
- 1 egg yolk
- 1 tablespoon of potato starch

Peel and grate one small carrot on a small plastic grater, add 1 tablespoon of cream, whipped yolk and 1 tablespoon of potato starch. Apply this mixture to your face for 15-20 minutes, then wash it off with cool water. This mask is useful for mature skin, it freshens and smoothes it.

✔ Carrot-apple mask

- 1 tablespoon of fresh apple pulp
- 1 tablespoon of carrot, grated

Mix 1 tablespoon of fresh apple pulp with 1 tablespoon of carrot grated on a small plastic grater. Put the mask on your face, leave for 20 minutes, then wash it off with cool water. This mask moistens and nourishes withering skin.

✔ Apple mask

- 1 baked apple
- Half a teaspoon of olive oil
- 1 teaspoon of honey

Add half a teaspoon of olive oil and 1 teaspoon of honey to the pulp of baked apple. Stir well and apply this mask to your face. In 15-20 minutes wash it off with warm, then with cool water. This mask freshens loose skin well and prevents its ageing.

✔ Banana and cream mask

- Slice of banana

- Warm cream

Knead a slice of banana, stir in the cream and apply to your face for 20 minutes. Wash it off with warm, then with cool water. If your skin is oily add some drops of lemon juice into this mixture. This mask smoothes and softens skin well.

✔ Egg-lemon mask

- 1 egg white
- 1 teaspoon of lemon juice
- Half a tablespoon of oatmeal

Whip the egg white, 1 teaspoon of lemon juice and half a tablespoon of oatmeal. Apply this mixture to your face and leave for 20 minutes. Wash it off with warm, then with cold water. This mask tones and bleaches withering skin and narrows pores well.

✔ Quince mask

- 1 tablespoon of quince
- 1 tablespoon of cream or egg white

Mix 1 tablespoon of quince grated on a small grater with 1 tablespoon of cream (for dry skin) or whipped egg white (for oily porous skin). Apply this mixture to your face and leave for 20-30 minutes. Then remove with a wet cotton wool ball and rinse the face with cool water. This mask clears, freshens and tones withering wrinkled skin.

✔ Apricot mask

- Ripe apricots
- 1 tablespoon of fresh sour cream

Mix 2 tablespoons of ripe apricot pulp with 1 tablespoon of fresh sour cream. Apply the mask to your face and leave for 20 minutes. Wash it off with cool water. This mask is useful for dry withering skin, it nourishes and freshens it well, makes it more elastic and smoothes wrinkles.

✔ Peach mask

- Juice of one peach

- 1 tablespoon of milk

- Oatmeal

Mix the peach juice with 1 tablespoon of fresh milk and add oatmeal. Stir to the consistency of gruel. Apply the mask to your face, leave for 20-30 minutes. Then wash it off with cold water. It clears and freshens flabby withering skin well.

✔ Persimmon mask

- 1 ripe persimmon

- 1 egg yolk

- 1 tablespoon of honey

- 2 teaspoons of aloe juice

Knead the ripe persimmon and add the egg yolk, 1 tablespoon of honey and 2 teaspoons of aloe juice. Stir thoroughly, and put this mask on your face for 20 minutes. Wash it off with warm water. The mask has a perfect rejuvenating effect.

✔ Pomegranate mask

- 1 tablespoon of pomegranate juice

- 1 tablespoon of sour cream

Mix 1 tablespoon of pomegranate juice with 1 tablespoon of sour cream and apply this mixture to your face. Leave the mask for 10 minutes, then wash it off with warm water. This mask rejuvenates and freshens withering skin.

✔ Sea-buckthorn mask

- Sea-buckthorn berries

- 1 tablespoon of fresh curds or sour cream

Mix 2 tablespoons of mashed sea-buckthorn berries with 1 tablespoon of fresh curds or sour cream. Apply this mixture to your face for 15-20 minutes, wash it off first with warm, then with cold water. This mask nourishes, moistens and rejuvenates withering skin, narrows enlarged/widened pores.

✔ Grape mask 1

- 1 egg white

- Grape pulp

- Grape juice

Whip the egg white into froth and add 1 tablespoon of mashed grape pulp. Spread your face with grape juice and apply the mask. Leave for 10-15 minutes. Then wash it off with cold water. This mask is useful for oily wrinkled skin.

✔ Grape mask 2

- Grape pulp

- 1 tablespoon of honey

Mix1 tablespoon of mashed grape pulp with 1 tablespoon of honey and apply this mixture to your face for 10-15 minutes. Wash this mask off with warm water. It is useful for dry withering skin.

✔ Grape mask 3

- Grape juice

- Fresh milk

Mix grape juice and fresh milk in equal parts. Moisten a napkin in this mixture and put it on your face. Leave the mask for 15-20 minutes and wash it off with some water. This mask is recommended for dry wrinkled skin. After this procedure it is useful to spread skin with a nourishing cream.

✔ **Grape mask 4**

- 1-1.5 tablespoons of grape juice

Moisten a linen or gauze napkin folded into several layers in grape juice, put it on your face for 10-15 minutes. After you remove it, rinse your face with warm water, wipe with a soft towel and apply some nourishing cream. A course comprises 15-20 procedures. The mask makes skin velvety, fresh and elastic, prevents flabbiness, clears and tones well.

✔ **Black currant mask**

- Ripe black currants

- 1 teaspoon of honey

Mix 1 tablespoon of kneaded ripe black currants with 1 teaspoon of honey and apply this mixture to the face. Leave the mask for 15 minutes. Wash it off with cool water. It tones withering skin well and bleaches it.

✔ **Red currant mask**

- Red currants

- 2 tablespoons of kefir or sour cream

Mix 1 tablespoon of red currant gruel with 2 tablespoons of kefir or sour cream. Apply to your face, then wash it off in 15-20 minutes. The mask is suitable for dry, withering, pigmented skin, and skin that has lost freshness.

✔ **Ashberry mask**

- Red ashberries

- 1 teaspoon of honey

- 1 teaspoon of hot water

Blend 2 tablespoons of kneaded red ashberries with 1 teaspoon of honey and 1 teaspoon of hot water. Apply this warm mixture to your face and leave for 20-30 minutes. Then wash it off with warm water. Ashberries rejuvenates skin well.

✔ Mask with mint and rosemary

- Half a tablespoon of crushed peppermint leaves

- Half a tablespoon of crushed rosemary leaves

- 400 ml of boiling water

- Starch

- 1 cube of mint ice

Add half a tablespoon of crushed peppermint and rosemary leaves to 100 ml of boiling water, cover and leave to infuse for 30 minutes. Then filter and add some starch into this infusion to the consistency of thick sour cream. Apply the mask to your face and leave for 20-30 minutes. Then wash it off with cool water and wipe your skin with a cube of mint ice. This mask calms and freshens withering skin and smoothes early wrinkles.

✔ Nettle mask

- 1 tablespoon of fresh kneaded nettle leaves

- 1 tablespoon of honey

Mix 1 tablespoon of fresh kneaded nettle leaves with 1 tablespoon of honey. Put the mask on your face for 10-15 minutes. Wash it off with warm, then with cold water. This mask is recommended for dry withering skin.

✔ Dandelion and plantain mask

- Fresh leaves of dandelion

- Fresh leaves of common plantain

- 1 teaspoon of cream

- 1 tablespoon of honey

- Olive oil

Add 1 teaspoon of cream to 1 tablespoon of crushed and kneaded fresh leaves of dandelion and common plantain and mix with 1 tablespoon of honey. Apply this mixture to your face, having greased it with olive oil first. Leave the mask for 10-15 minutes. Wash it off with warm, then with cold water. This mask moistens, nourishes and rejuvenates withering skin.

✓ **Herbal mask 1**

- 1 tablespoon of chamomile flowers

- 1 tablespoon of linden flowers

- 1 tablespoon of lavender flowers

- 1 tablespoon of crushed hop cones

- 1 tablespoon of birch leaves

- Boiling water

Add 1 tablespoon of each ingredient (chamomile flowers, linden flowers, lavender flowers, crushed, hop cones, birch leaves) to some boiling water. Let it infuse for few minutes, apply this warm mixture to your face and leave for 15 minutes. Wash it off with water. This mask rejuvenates withering skin.

✓ **Herbal mask 2**

- Nettle leaves

- Mint leaves

- Leaves of black currant

- Raspberry leaves

- 1 tablespoon of curds

- 1 teaspoon of honey

Blend 1 tablespoon of crushed leaves of nettle, mint, black currant, raspberry with 1 tablespoon of curds and 1 teaspoon of honey. Apply this mixture to your face for 20 minutes. Then wash it off with warm water. This mask moistens, nourishes and rejuvenates dry withering skin.

✔ Herbal mask 3

- Sage leaves

- Common wormwood herb

- Yarrow herb

- Water

Mix crushed leaves of sage, common wormwood herb and yarrow in equal parts. Add 2 tablespoons of this mixture to a fair amount of water, bring to a boil, remove from the heat and let it infuse. Then filter and put the herbal mask on your face. Leave the mask for15 minutes and wash it off with a herbal tincture. This mask is useful for oily withering skin with nlarged/widened pores.

✔ Mask with mustard

- Half a teaspoon of mustard powder

- Half a tablespoon of tutsan herb

- 200 ml of water

- 1 teaspoon of melted butter

To prepare the tutsan extract add half a tablespoon of tutsan herb to 200 ml of water, heat on a water bath for 30 minutes, then filter. Dissolve half a teaspoon of mustard powder in 5 tablespoons of warm tutsan extract, add 1 teaspoon of melted butter. Apply this mixture to your face with a cotton wool ball. Leave the mask for few minutes depending on sensitivity of skin, then wash it off with cool water, directing the shower stream to your face. After that apply nourishing cream to the face. Apply this mask once a week. The mask is suitable for wrinkled flabby skin.

✔ Grapefruit mask

- 2 tablespoons of grapefruit juice

- 1 tablespoon of rice flour

- 1 tablespoon of sour cream

Mix tablespoons of grapefruit juice with 1 tablespoon of rice flour and 1 tablespoon of sour cream. Such masks smooth wrinkles and prevent their occurrence.

✔ Crisphead lettuce mask

- Leaves of crisphead lettuce

- Olive oil

- 1 teaspoon of lemon juice

Chop and knead the leaves of crisphead lettuce and mix with olive oil and lemon juice. Apply this mixture to your face for 20 minutes, then remove with a cotton wool ball and wash the face with warm water at first, then with cold water. This mask freshens calloused, dry, withering skin.

✔ Sour cream mask with tea

- 2 teaspoons of dried small-leaved green tea

- Boiling water

- 1 tablespoon of thick sour cream

Brew small-leaved green tea with a little of boiling water for 2-3 minutes and pour the liquid out. Mix 1 tablespoon of thick sour cream with stewed tea and put the mask on your face. In 15-20 minutes wash the mask off with warm water and apply some nourishing cream.

✓ Mask with tea butter

- 3–4 drops of tea butter
- 1 tablespoon of thick sour cream
- Half a teaspoon of apricot pulp or grated fresh cucumber
- 1 cube of herbal infusion ice

Mix 1 tablespoon of thick sour cream with half a teaspoon of apricot pulp or fresh cucumber grated on a small grater, add 3-4 drops of tea butter. Stir carefully and apply to your face. In 30 minutes wash the mask off with warm water, and then wipe the skin with a cube of herbal infusion ice: chamomile, calendula, parsley and mint. This mask with tea butter will help to tone tired, withering skin.

✓ Lemon mask

- 1 egg yolk
- 1 teaspoon of honey
- 1 teaspoon of vegetable oil
- 1 teaspoon of lemon juice

Mix the egg yolk, 2 teaspoons of honey, 1 teaspoon of vegetable oil and1 teaspoon of lemon juice. Apply this mixture to your face for 15-20 minutes, wash it off with cool water. The mask is useful for dry, dehydrated and withering skin.

✓ Carrot-lemon mask

- 1 tablespoon of lemon juice
- 1 tablespoon of carrot juice
- 1 tablespoon of curdled milk
- 1 tablespoon of rice flour

Mix 1 tablespoon of lemon juice, carrot juice, curdled milk and rice flour and apply to your face two to three times a week. A course comprises 20 procedures.

✓ Milk-apple mask

- 1 tablespoon of ripe apple, grated

- 40 ml of cream or milk

- 1 egg white (for oily skin)

Grate one juicy ripe apple. Add a tablespoon of the apple pulp to 40 ml of boiling cream or milk, boil for 2-3 minutes, then leave to infuse for 30 minutes. If you have oily skin, add a whipped egg white to this mixture. Apply it to the face and neck for 20-30 minutes, then wash it off with cool water. This procedure freshens and rejuvenates skin.

✓ Wild strawberry mask

- 50 ml of milk

- 50 ml of wild strawberry juice

Mix 50 ml of milk and 50 ml of strawberry juice. Put a layer of cotton wool moistened in this mixture on your face for 15-20 minutes, covered with a towel. After removal of this mask wipe the skin carefully and apply a nourishing cream.

Creams for withering facial skin

✓ Cream with aloe

- 30 g of lanolin cream

- 1 tablespoon of olive oil

- 1 tablespoon of biostimulating aloe juice

- Herbal infusion

Mix 30 g of lanolin cream with 1 tablespoon of olive oil and 1 tablespoon of biostimulating aloe juice. Warm this mixture on a water bath and apply to the skin of your face and neck while it is warm. After 20 minutes remove the remains of the cream with a cotton wool ball moistened in herbal infusion (sage, rosemary, mint or chamomile) and rinse the face with the infusion.

✓ Cream with cocoa butter

- 10 g of beeswax
- 10 g of cocoa butter
- 25 ml of distilled water
- 0.5 g of borax
- 3 drops of geranium essential oil
- 2 drops of rose or lavender essential oil

Melt 10 g of beeswax and 10 g of cocoa butter on a water bath and stir thoroughly, gradually adding 25 ml of distilled water. At the end add a small amount of borax crystals (0.5 g). Cool this cream to room temperature, stir again and add 3 drops of geranium essential oil and 2 drops of rose or lavender essential oil. This cream smoothes small wrinkles and is recommended for mature skin. Store it in a refrigerator for no more than two weeks in a tightly sealed vessel.

✓ Lemon cream

- 1 lemon
- 200 ml of boiling water
- 1 tablespoon of cream
- 1 teaspoon of honey
- 1 teaspoon of wheat sprout oil
- 20 ml of vodka
- 50 ml of rose petal infusion (2 tablespoons of petals, 200 ml of boiling water)

Squeeze out 1 lemon. Crush lemon peel, add 200 ml of boiling water and leave to infuse in a warm place for 2 hours. Then filter, add lemon juice, 1 tablespoon of cream, 2 teaspoons of honey, 1 teaspoon of wheat sprout oil, 20 ml of vodka, 50 ml of rose petal infusion and stir thoroughly. This cream is useful for withering old skin. Apply it to your face and neck before sleep, then after 20 minutes remove the remains with a napkin.

✔ Honey cream with white lily juice

- 25 g of beeswax
- 1 tablespoon of vegetable oil
- 2 tablespoons of honey
- 2 teaspoons of white lily bulb juice

Melt 25 g of beeswax on a water bath, add 1 tablespoon of vegetable oil, 2 tablespoons of honey and 2 teaspoons of white lily bulb juice. Stir thoroughly and let it cool down. Apply as a night cream. It prevents skin aging, smoothing small wrinkles.

✔ Yolk cream with chamomile

- 1 egg yolk
- 25 g of fresh butter
- Half a tablespoon of chamomile infusion (3 tablespoons of chamomile flowers, 200 ml of water)
- Half a teaspoon of honey
- 1 teaspoon of glycerin
- 1 tablespoon of camphor spirit

Knead the egg yolk with 25 g of fresh butter, add half a tablespoon of chamomile infusion (add 3 tablespoons of chamomile flowers to 200 ml of water, heat on a water bath for 15 minutes and leave to infuse at room temperature for 45 minutes), half a teaspoon of honey, 1 teaspoon of glycerin and 1 tablespoon of camphor spirit and stir thoroughly. This cream is recommended for dry wrinkled skin.

✔ Persimmon cream

- Half a ripe persimmon
- 1 egg yolk
- 1 teaspoon of honey
- 1 teaspoon of sea-buckthorn juice
- 1 teaspoon of aloe juice
- 30 g of a nourishing cream

Mix the pulp of persimmon with the egg yolk, 1 teaspoon of honey, 1 teaspoon of sea-buckthorn juice, 1 teaspoon of aloe juice and 30 g of any nourishing cream. This cream nourishes and moistens tired skin, helping with first signs of aging.

✔ Nourishing cream with herbs

- Fresh nettle leaves
- Fresh parsley leaves
- Fresh currant leaves
- Jasmine petals
- Rose petals
- 10 g of beeswax
- 50 g of fresh butter
- 1 tablespoon of vegetable oil
- 1 teaspoon of vitamin A oil solution

Mince the fresh nettle, parsley, currant and jasmine leaves along with rose petals taken in equal parts. Melt 10 g of beeswax and 50 g of fresh butter on a water bath and add 1 tablespoon of vegetable oil. Then add 1 teaspoon of vitamin A oil solution and 1 tablespoon of herbal mixture and stir everything thoroughly. Use this cream for dry withering skin.

✔ White lily cream

- 30 g of beeswax

- 2 tablespoons of white lily bulb juice

- 2 tablespoons of onion juice

Melt 30 g of beeswax on a water bath, add 2 tablespoons of white lily bulb juice and 2 tablespoons of onion juice. Stir well and let it cool down. Apply this cream to your face in the morning and in the evening. It smoothes wrinkles, making skin smooth and elastic.

Skin care recipes for problem-prone facial skin

Problem-prone facial skin (p.176)

Problem-prone facial skin inclined to irritation and inflammation cleansing (p.176)

Infusions and lotions for problem-prone facial skin inclined to irritation and inflammation (p.178)

Masks for problem-prone facial skin inclined to irritation and inflammation (p.181)

Tinctures for acne skin care (p.186)

Plant extracts, tinctures and juices for acne skin care (p.187)

Lotions for acne skin care (p.192)

Compresses for acne skin care (p.196)

Masks for acne skin care (p.199)

Compresses for facial skin with acne rosacea (p.203)

Masks for facial skin with acne rosacea (p.204)

Tinctures, infusions and decoctions for bleaching facial skin with pigment spots and freckles (p.207)

Lotions for facial skin with pigment spots and freckles (p.209)

Bleaching masks for facial skin with pigment spots and freckles (p.211)

Bleaching creams for facial skin with pigment spots and freckles (p.219)

Sunburn protection (p.220)

Compresses on sunburns (p.222)

Masks on sunburns (p.224)

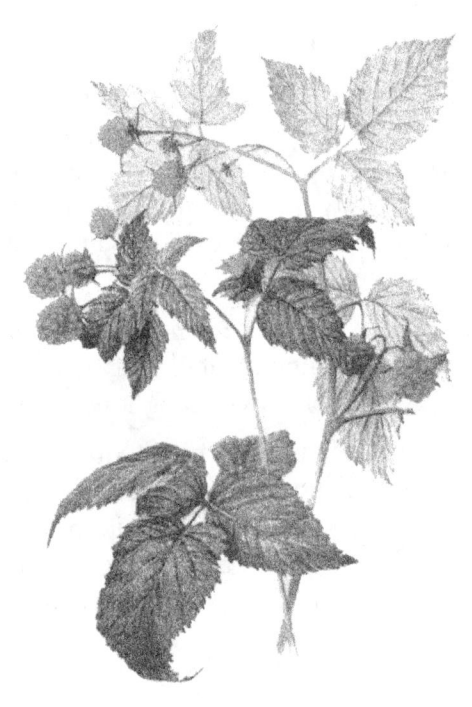

Problem-prone facial skin

Problem-prone skin is called such for having a number of defects: rashes, inflammations, impure pores, pigment spots or scars.

Problem-prone skin care basically consists of cleansing impure enlarged pores.

Make sure to wash your face with neutral soap. Before washing, it is useful to apply lactoserum, kefir or thick sour milk on your skin and to add lemon juice to the water used for washing (1 teaspoon per 1 liter of water).

After washing it is necessary to use cleansing, disinfectant, astringent lotions, extracts and tinctures of various medicinal grasses which possess astringent and drying properties. A little bit of vodka or cologne may be added to these infusions, so they can be used as toilet water. It is useful to wipe the face with a cube of ice made of some herbal decoction.

If problem-prone skin is dry, irritated and peels under the influence of products containing alcohol, it should be cleansed with cosmetic milk and softened with a light nourishing cream.

Problem-prone skin is effectively cleansed with the help of peelings and masks containing organic acids or enzymes, which dissolve dead cells and moisturize skin, ensuring its healthy appearance. Clay masks and steam baths are very effective. The main aspect of problem-prone skin care is the regularity of procedures.

Problem-prone facial skin inclined to irritation and inflammation cleansing

✓ **Corn-almond flour**

- 3 tablespoons of corn flour

- 1 tablespoon of sweet almond flour

- Hot water

Mix 3 tablespoons of corn flour and 1 tablespoon of sweet almond flour with hot water to the consistency of gruel. Use this mix for dry sensitive skin cleansing. Apply to the face for 10-15 minutes, then wash it off with warm water.

✔ Potato starch

- Potato starch

Mix starch with water, wrap in a gauze napkin and massage the face with it. Potato starch is a soft natural scrub for dry sensitive skin which not only cleanses well but also bleaches.

✔ Rice peeling

- 1 glass of rice flour

- 1 teaspoon of baking soda

- Yoghurt

Add 1 teaspoon of baking soda to a glass of rice flour, stir well and store in tightly sealed glass jar. For facial cleansing dilute 1 tablespoon of this mixture with yoghurt to the consistency of gruel. Put it on your face with a cotton wool ball, massaging skin with circular movements. In 2-3 minutes wash it off with warm water. This procedure clears and rejuvenates oily skin with acne punctata.

✔ Egg yolk with vegetable oil

- 1 egg yolk

- 1 tablespoon of vegetable oil

- 1 tablespoon of water

If your sensitive dry skin is intolerant of soap, apply 1 whipped egg yolk, mixed with 1 tablespoon of vegetable oil and 1 tablespoon of water. Wash it off with warm water after 10 minutes.

✓ Viburnum juice

- Viburnum juice

In the morning after washing the face with warm water, wipe oily problem-prone skin with a cube of viburnum juice ice (you can also use raspberry, strawberry, cowberry or cranberry juices).

✓ Emulsion instead of washing

- Cucumber juice

- 1 egg yolk

- Half a glass of cream

- 1 tablespoon of vodka

For irritated dry skin wipe the face with the following emulsion instead of washing: mix cucumber juice with the egg yolk, half a glass of cream and 1 tablespoon of vodka, stir everything thoroughly, filter and store in a glass bottle in a cool place.

Infusions and lotions for problem-prone facial skin inclined to irritation and inflammation

✓ Peony (Paeonia anomala) infusion

- 1 tablespoon of crushed peony root (Paeonia anomala)

- 250 ml of water

Add 1 tablespoon of crushed peony root to 250 ml of water, cover and heat on a water bath for 15 minutes, let it infuse for 45 minutes and filter. In the case of skin inflammation apply compresses moistened in this infusion to your face.

✓ Melissa tincture

- 1 tablespoon of melissa leaves

- 200 ml of water

Add 1 tablespoon of melissa leaves to 200 ml of water, heat on a water bath for 15 minutes, then let it infuse at room temperature for 45 minutes and filter. Wipe overly sensitive skin inclined to irritation with this infusion instead of washing.

✔ Tutsan and chamomile decoction

- 1 tablespoon of tutsan herb
- Half a tablespoon of chamomile flowers
- 200 ml of water

Combine 1 tablespoon of tutsan herb and 0,5 tablespoon of chamomile flowers with 200 ml of water, heat on a water bath for 30 minutes, filter and cool down for 10 minutes. This decoction freshens and calms problem-prone skin.

✔ Poppy tincture

- 5-7 poppy flowers
- 250 ml of boiling water
- Half a teaspoon of honey

Add 5-7 field poppy flowers to 250 ml of boiling water, add half a teaspoon of honey, cover and leave to infuse for 10-15 minutes. Then filter and use to wipe the face in the morning to help against irritation, dryness, redness and skin eruption.

✔ Plantain lotion

- Fresh plantain leaves
- Vodka

Crush fresh plantain leaves, wring the juice out and add vodka (4:1). Wipe inflamed irritated oily skin with this lotion. Store in a dark, cool place.

✓ Lemon lotion

- 1 lemon
- 100 ml of water
- 1 teaspoon of glycerin

Grate the lemon with rind on a grater, add 100 ml of cold water and leave to infuse in a dark place for a week. Then filter, wring out the rest of the raw material and add 1 teaspoon of glycerin to the tincture. Use this lotion for cleansing oily problem-prone skin.

✓ Rose lotion 1

- 1 handful of fresh rose petals
- 100 ml of boiled water
- 1 teaspoon of honey
- 5 drops of lemon juice

Add 1 handful of fresh rose petals to 100 ml of boiled water and let it infuse for 20-30 minutes. Filter this infusion and add 1 teaspoon of honey and 5 drops of lemon juice. Stir thoroughly and apply this mixture to your previously cleared face with a cotton wool ball, leave for 10-15 minutes, then wash it off with cool water. This lotion alleviates inflammation and freshens skin.

✓ Rose lotion 2

- 1 handful of dried rose petals
- 100 ml of tea mushroom infusion
- 70 ml of mineral water

Add 1 handful of dried rose petals to 100 ml of tea mushroom infusion, add 70 ml of mineral water and leave to infuse in a dark, cool place for two weeks in a tightly sealed vessel, then filter. Wipe oily skin inclined to inflammation in the morning and in the evening with this lotion.

✓ Flower lotion

- Dried rose petals
- Linden flowers
- Nasturtium flowers
- Bluebottle flowers
- 200 ml of boiling water
- 1 teaspoon of lemon juice

Mix the crushed rose petals, linden flowers, nasturtium flowers and bluebottle flowers taken in equal parts. Add 1 tablespoon of this mix to 200 ml of boiling water, let it infuse for 2 hours, filter and add 1 teaspoon of lemon juice. Wipe sensitive skin inclined to irritation in the morning and in the evening with this lotion.

✓ Watermelon and cucumber lotion

- 50 ml of watermelon juice
- 50 ml of cucumber juice

Mix 50 ml of watermelon juice and 50 ml of cucumber juice. Use this lotion in case of redness of your facial skin.

Masks for problem-prone skin inclined to irritation and inflammation

✓ Calming mask with spinach

- 4-5 spinach leaves
- 1 glass of milk

Wash 4-5 spinach leaves carefully, crush and boil in 1 glass of milk. Put them on a gauze napkin and apply this mask to the face and neck. Remove after 15-20 minutes. Wipe your skin with this lotion and apply some moisturizing cream. The mask not only calms irritated skin but also possesses cleansing and freshening properties.

✓ **Honey-milk mask**

- 1 teaspoon of honey

- 1 teaspoon of milk

- 1 teaspoon of potato starch

- 1 teaspoon of salt

Mix 1 teaspoon of honey with 1 teaspoon of milk and add 1 teaspoon of potato starch and 1 teaspoon of salt. Stir well and apply this mixture to your face. Leave the mask for 20 minutes, then wash it off first with warm water, then with cool water. This mask is useful for oily skin with enlarged pores inclined to inflammation.

✓ **Egg-corn mask**

- 1 tablespoon of corn flour

- 1 egg white

Mix 1 tablespoon of corn flour with the whipped egg white. After it dries remove the mask with a dry linen napkin and rinse the face with cold water.

✓ **Potato mask**

- Potato

Grate raw potato on a grater and put this mask on your face. Leave for 15-20 minutes, then wash it off with warm water. This mask clears skin well, eliminating redness and skin eruption.

✓ **Pear mask**

- 1 ripe pear, pulped

- 1 teaspoon of rice or corn starch

- 1 teaspoon of lemon juice

Mix pear pulp with1 teaspoon of rice or corn starch and 1 teaspoon of lemon juice. Apply this mask to your face, leave for 15-20 minutes, then wash it off with cool water. This mask clears problem-prone skin well.

✔ Strawberry mask

- 2 teaspoons of kneaded strawberries

- 2 teaspoons of honey

- 1 teaspoon of curds

Mix 2 teaspoons of kneaded strawberries with 2 teaspoons of honey and1 teaspoon of fresh curds. Apply this mixture to your face. Leave the mask for 10-15 minutes. Then wash it off with warm water and rinse the face with cool water. This mask clears and nourishes sensitive skin.

✔ Fireweed mask with oat flakes

- Ground oat flakes

- Pinch of salt

- Fireweed tincture (3 tablespoonfuls of fireweed (Epilobium angustifolium), 250 ml of vodka)

Mix 20 ml of fireweed tincture with ground oat flakes and salt to the consistency of gruel and apply this mask to your preliminarily cleansed face. Leave the mask for15 minutes, then wash it off with cool water. Repeat this procedure daily or every other day. It alleviates skin inflammation and has a toning effect. To prepare the fireweed tincture take 3 tablespoons of crushed crops and add 250 ml of vodka, leave to infuse in a dark place for three weeks, then filter.

✔ Raspberry mask

- Fresh raspberry leaves

Put finely cut fresh raspberry leaves on your face, having applied a nourishing cream first. Leave the mask for 10-15 minutes. This mask alleviates skin inflammation and tones skin.

✓ **Compress with chamomile infusion**

- 4 tablespoons of chamomile flowers

- 200 ml of water

Add 4 tablespoons of chamomile flowers to 200 ml of hot water, heat on a water bath for 15 minutes, let it infuse at room temperature for 45 minutes and filter. Moisten a napkin in the warm infusion, wring it out slightly and apply to your face. Leave for five minutes. Repeat this procedure several times. In case of oily skin inclined to inflammation apply compresses daily for 10-12 days.

✓ **Tea compress**

- Tea brew

Moisten a gauze or linen napkin in a fresh tea brew and, having wrung it out slightly, apply to the face for 15-20 minutes. If the skin is dry, apply a nourishing cream after the compress. This compress is effective against irritated skin with enlarged pores.

✓ **Kefir mask**

- 2 tablespoons of kefir

- 1 teaspoon of wheat sprout oil

- 1 egg yolk

Mix 2 tablespoons of kefir with 1 teaspoon of wheat sprout oil and 1 whipped egg yolk. Apply a thin layer of this mask to your face. Leave for 20 minutes and wash it off with warm milk. This mask is recommended for dry inflamed skin that peels.

✔ Cucumber-almond mask

- 1 tablespoon of cucumber juice

- 1 tablespoon of almond oil

Mix 1 tablespoon of cucumber juice and almond oil, moisten a gauze napkin in this mix and apply to the face. Leave this mask for 20-30 minutes, then wash it off with warm water and rinse the face with cold water. This mask makes skin soft and velvety. It is useful against calluses and chapped skin.

✔ Apple mask

- 1 apple

- 1 egg yolk

- 1 tablespoon of fresh milk

Peel the apple and grate on a small plastic grater, add the egg yolk and1 tablespoon of fresh milk and stir thoroughly. Apply this mixture to your face, leave for 20 minutes and wash it off with soft warm water. This mask is useful for sensitive skin inclined to redness.

✔ Rose petal mask

- Powdered dried rose petals

- 2 tablespoons of natural yoghurt or sour cream

- Rose water

Mix 1 tablespoon of rose petals with 2 tablespoons of natural yoghurt (for oily skin) or sour cream (for dry skin) and apply this mixture to the cleansed skin of your face. Leave the mask for 20-30 minutes then remove with a napkin and wipe the face with a cotton wool ball moistened in rose water. This mask nourishes, softens and tones skin.

✔ Curds, sour cream and egg white mask

- Half a glass of curds

- Sour cream

- 1 egg white

This mask is very useful for inflamed or irritated skin. Mix half a glass of curds with a small amount of sour cream and a whipped egg white until you get a thick gruel. Apply this mask to your skin for 15-20 minutes.

Tinctures for acne skin care

✔ Raspberry leaf tincture

- 40 g of raspberry leaves

- 200 ml of vodka

Add 40 g of raspberry leaves to 200 ml of vodka, leave to infuse in a dark place for 2 weeks, filter and wipe acne-prone skin with this tincture.

✔ Raspberry tincture

- 1 tablespoon of raspberries

- 250 ml of vodka

- Distilled water

Knead 1 tablespoon of raspberries and add 250 ml of vodka. Leave to infuse in a dark place for 10 days and filter. Before application dilute with distilled water at a 1:1 ratio.

✔ Bluebottle tincture

- 40 g of bluebottle flowers

- 200 ml of vodka

- Water

Add 40 g of bluebottle marginal flowers to 200 ml of vodka and leave to infuse in a dark place for 2 weeks. Then filter this tincture, dilute with water at a 1:1 ratio and use to wipe oily skin with acne.

✔ White lily tincture

- White lily petals

- Vodka

Fill a half-liter bottle with white lily petals, pour vodka over them and leave to infuse in a dark place for 2 weeks, then filter and wipe your skin for the night. This tincture is one of the best means for acne treatment.

✔ Rose petal tincture

- Fresh rose petals

- Vodka

Fill a half-liter bottle with fresh rose petals, pour vodka over to the brim and leave to infuse in a dark place for 2 weeks, stirring daily. Then filter and store in a tightly sealed vessel. Wipe oily skin with this tincture. It possesses astringent and antiseptic properties, preventing and treating pustular eruptions.

Plant extracts, tinctures and juices for acne skin care

✔ Haricot infusion

- 3 tablespoons of chamomile flowers

- 100 g of haricot

- Half a liter of boiled water

To prepare the extract add 100 g of haricot to half a liter of boiled water and boil on a low heat for 30 minutes. Add 3 tablespoons of chamomile flowers to 200 ml of the hot extract, leave to infuse until it cools down and then filter it. Rinse your face with this extract 3 times a day in case of chronic acne.

✔ Nettle tincture

- 1 tablespoon of great nettle leaves
- 200 ml of boiling water

Add 1 tablespoon of great nettle leaves to 200 ml of boiling water, leave to infuse for 30 minutes and filter. Rinse your face with this infusion 5-6 times a day to help care for oily skin and acne.

✔ Pine extract

- Buds, young cones or pine needles
- Water

Add crushed buds, young cones or pine needles to water at a 1:5 ratio, boil on a low heat in a closed pot for 30 minutes, let it cool down and filter. Rinse your face with this extract when acne is present.

✔ Bird cherry leaves and flowers infusion

- 4 tablespoons of bird cherry leaves and flowers
- 200 ml of boiling water

Add 4 tablespoons of bird cherry leaves and flowers to 200 ml of boiling water, leave to infuse for 30 minutes, filter and rinse your face with this infusion.

✔ Elecampane rhizome extract

- 1 tablespoon of crushed elecampane rhizomes
- 200 ml of water

Add 1 tablespoon of crushed elecampane rhizomes to 200 ml of water, heat on a water bath for 30 minutes, let it cool down for 10 minutes and filter. Use this extract for washing your face.

✔ Oak bark extract

- 2 tablespoons of oak bark
- 200 ml of water

Add 2 tablespoons of oak bark to 200 ml of water, heat on a water bath for 30 minutes, filter and let it cool down. Wipe oily skin with enlarged pores and acne with this extract.

✔ Oak bark and tutsan extract

- 1 tablespoon of oak bark
- 1 tablespoon of tutsan herb
- 200 ml of boiling water
- Cool water

Add 1 tablespoon of oak bark and tutsan to 200 ml of boiling water, boil for 10 minutes, leave to infuse for 20 minutes, filter and add cool water to the initial volume. This extract is recommended for facial wiping for those with excessive sebaceous excretions.

✔ White willow bark extract

- 1 tablespoon of crushed white willow bark
- 200 ml of boiling water

Add 1 tablespoon of crushed white willow bark to 200 ml of boiling water, boil for 10 minutes on a low heat, filter and let it cool down. Rinse your face with this extract.

✔ Tutsan extract

- 1.5 tablespoons of tutsan

- 200 ml of water

Add 1.5 tablespoons of tutsan herb to 200 ml of water, heat on a water bath for 30 minutes, filter and let it cool down at room temperature for 10 minutes. Use for wiping skin with acne.

✔ **Horsetail extract**

- 4 tablespoons of field horsetail

- 200 ml of water

Add 4 tablespoons of field horsetail to 200 ml of water, heat on a water bath for 30 minutes, let it cool down for 10 minutes and filter. Use for wiping inflamed skin with acne.

✔ **Serpent grass extract**

- 2 teaspoons of crushed serpent grass rhizome

- 200 ml of water

Add 2 teaspoons of crushed serpent grass rhizome to 200 ml of water, heat on a water bath for 30 minutes, filter, let it cool down and wipe your face with the extract.

✔ **Marshmallow root tincture**

- 3 tablespoons of crushed marshmallow root

- Half a liter of cool water

Add 3 tablespoons of crushed marshmallow root to half a liter of cool water and leave to infuse for 8 hours. Filter and use for wiping skin with acne and in the creation of lotions and compresses.

✔ **Bur-marigold herb tincture**

- 3 tablespoons of crushed bur-marigold herb

- 200 ml of water

Add 3 tablespoons of crushed bur-marigold herb to 200 ml of water, heat on a water bath for 15 minutes, leave to infuse at room temperature for 45 minutes, filter and wipe your skin with the infusion.

✓ Raspberry leaves extract

- 2 tablespoons of raspberry leaves

- 250 ml of water

Add 2 tablespoons of raspberry leaves to 250 ml of water, boil on a low heat for 5-7 minutes, let it cool down, filter and wipe your face. This infusion clears skin well and makes it elastic.

✓ Aloe leaves infusion

- 40 g of kneaded biostimulating aloe leaves

- 200 ml of cool water

Add 40 g of kneaded biostimulating aloe leaves to 200 ml of cool water, leave to infuse for an hour, then bring to the boil on a low heat, boil for 2-3 minutes and let it cool down. Filter and use for wiping the face and in lotions for inflamed skin and acne.

✓ Aloe juice

- Biostimulating aloe leaves

Wring the juice out of biostimulating aloe leaves and wipe your skin 2-3 times a day to battle acne. Aloe juice helps alleviate irritation and skin inflammation.

✓ Viburnum juice

- Fresh viburnum juice

Wipe oily porous skin with acne with fresh viburnum juice 2-3 times a day.

✔ Strawberry juice

- Fresh strawberry juice

Wipe your face with fresh strawberry juice 2-3 times a day for acne treatment.

✔ Stone bramble, bog bilberry and cloudberry leaves juice

- Stone bramble, bog bilberry and cloudberry leaves juice

Spread this juice upon skin zones troubled by acne.

✔ Plantain juice

- Plantain juice

Apply this juice to oily skin with acne vulgaris in the morning and in the evening. It eliminates inflammation and narrows pores.

✔ Birch sap

- Birch sap

Rinse your face with birch sap if you have oily skin with acne.

✔ Tomato juice

- Tomato juice

Clean your face then wipe it with fresh tomato juice or a slice of tomato to help alleviate acne.

Lotions for acne skin care

✓ Lemon (orange) lotion

- 1 lemon or orange
- Cool water
- 1 teaspoon of glycerin

Grate 1 lemon or 1 orange with rind and add 100 ml of cool water. Leave to infuse in a dark place for 5-7 days, then filter and wring out the remains of the raw material. Add 1 tablespoon of water and 1 teaspoon of glycerin to the infusion. Use this lotion for cleansing oily problem-prone skin.

✓ Strawberry lotion

- Strawberry juice
- Glycerin

Use strawberry juice with glycerin (at a 3:1 proportion) for wiping oily porous skin with acne. After 15 minutes rinse your face with warm water.

✓ Watermelon and cucumber lotion

- 50 ml of watermelon juice
- 50 ml of cucumber juice
- 50 ml of vodka

Mix 50 ml of watermelon juice with 50 ml of cucumber juice and add 50 ml of vodka. This lotion is highly effective against acne.

✓ Cucumber lotion 1

- 1 cucumber
- 200 ml of boiling water
- 1 teaspoon of honey

Peel 1 cucumber and grate on a small plastic grater. Add 3 tablespoons of cucumber mass to 200 ml of boiling water and leave to infuse for 2 hours. Then filter, wring out the remains of the raw material, add 1 teaspoon of honey and stir well. Wipe your skin with this lotion. After 30 minutes wash it off with cool water.

✔ Cucumber lotion 2

- 1 cucumber

- 100 ml of vodka

Chop 1 cucumber, add 100 ml of vodka, leave to infuse for 10 days in a tightly sealed vessel, then filter. This lotion can be stored in a refrigerator for 6 months.

✔ Grapefruit lotion

- 50 ml of grapefruit juice

- 50 ml of oak bark decoction (2 tablespoons of oak bark, 200 ml of water)

Mix 50 ml of grapefruit juice with 50 ml of oak bark extract (add 2 tablespoons of oak bark to 200 ml of water, heat on a water bath for 30 minutes, filter and let it cool) and wipe your face. This lotion is effective for acne treatment.

✔ Lotion with calendula

- 1 teaspoon of calendula tincture (40 g of calendula flowers, 200 ml of vodka)

- 200 ml of warm water

- 1 teaspoon of honey

Dilute 1 teaspoon of calendula tincture (add 40 g of calendula flowers to 200 ml of vodka, leave to infuse for 2 weeks and filter) to 200 ml of warm water, add 1 teaspoon of honey and stir. Wipe oily inflamed skin with this lotion 2-3 times a day.

✔ Sage lotion

- 1 tablespoon of sage leaves
- 200 ml of boiling water
- 1 teaspoon of honey

Add 1 tablespoon of sage leaves to 200 ml of boiling water, leave to infuse in a closed vessel for 30 minutes and filter. Add 1 teaspoon of honey to this infusion and stir well.Use this lotion for cleansing facial skin with acne.

✔ Tutsan and chamomile lotion

- 120 ml of tutsan extract (1.5 tablespoons of tutsan herb, water)
- 30 ml of chamomile tincture (4 tablespoons of chamomile flowers, water)
- 30 ml of vodka
- 10 ml of glycerin

Mix 120 ml of tutsan decoction (1.5 tablespoons of tutsan herb per 200 ml of water, boil), 30 ml of chamomile tincture (4 tablespoons of chamomile flowers per 200 ml of water, leave to infuse), 30 ml of vodka and 10 ml of glycerin. Use this lotion for cleansing oily skin with acne.

✔ Plantain lotion

- 1 tablespoon of common plantain juice
- 50 ml of vodka

Mix 1 tablespoon of common plantain juice with 50 ml of vodka and wipe your face in the morning and in the evening with this lotion if you have oily skin with acne.

✔ Hazel lotion

- 1 tablespoon of crushed hazel branches

- 200 ml of water

- 1 tablespoon of onion juice

To prepare the hazel extract add 1 tablespoon of crushed hazel branches to 200 ml of water, heat on a water bath in a closed vessel for 30 minutes and filter. Mix 100 ml of this extract with 1 tablespoon of onion juice. This lotion has antiseptic properties, perfect for cleansing oily skin.

✔ **Oak bark lotion for acne treatment**

- 2 tablespoons of dried crushed oak bark

- Half a liter of water

- Juice of a small grapefruit

- 2 tablespoons of vodka

Add 2 tablespoons of dried crushed oak bark to half a liter of water and boil for 5 minutes. Add the grapefruit juice and 2 tablespoons of vodka to the filtered extract. Wipe your cleansed face 2-3 times with a cotton wool ball moistened in this lotion. Then rinse the face with water. Use for acne, especially if pustules appear.

Compresses for acne skin care

For facial skin with acne apply warm compresses and change them continuously as they become cold.

✔ **Potato compress**

- 100 g of potato

- 1 teaspoon of honey

Add1 teaspoon of honey to 100 g of potato grated on a small grater and stir well. Put this mixture on a gauze napkin and cover the skin with it. Fix the compress and leave it on your face for 2 hours. This compress can be applied 2-3 times a day.

✔ Compress with raspberry leaf infusion

- 2 tablespoons of crushed raspberry leaves

- 200 ml of boiling water

Add 2 tablespoons of crushed raspberry leaves to 200 ml of boiling water, leave to infuse for 15-20 minutes in a closed vessel and filter. Moisten a napkin in this infusion, wring it out slightly and apply to your face. Leave the compress for 10 minutes. Repeat this procedure 3 times. A full course comprises 20-25 procedures. Apply compresses daily during the first half of the course, and every other day during the second.

✔ Compress with viburnum juice

- Viburnum juice

Moisten a gauze napkin in fresh viburnum juice and put it on your face. Leave the compress for 5-7 minutes, then change it 2-3 times with 10 minute breaks. After this procedure spread your face with a nourishing cream. A full course comprises 20 procedures. Do the first 10 procedures daily, and then every other day.

✔ Compress with birch infusion

- 1 tablespoon of birch buds

- 200 ml of water

Add 1 tablespoon of crushed birch buds to 200 ml of water and heat on a water bath for 15 minutes. Let it infuse for 45 minutes and filter. Use this infusion for acne skin care compresses.

✔ Compress with melissa infusion

- 2 tablespoons of melissa

- 200 ml of boiling water

Add 2 tablespoons of melissa to 200 ml of boiling water, leave to infuse for 1 hour and filter. Apply compresses with this warm infusion.

✔ Compress with wormwood infusion

- 2 tablespoons of common wormwood
- 300 ml of water

Add 2 tablespoons of common wormwood to 300 ml of water. Heat on a water bath for 15 minutes, let it infuse in a closed vessel for 45 minutes and filter. Use this infusion for compresses.

✔ Compress with chamomile infusion

- 2 tablespoons of chamomile flowers
- 200 ml of water

Add 2 tablespoons of chamomile flowers to 200 ml of water, heat on a water bath for 15 minutes, leave to infuse for 45 minutes and filter. Moisten napkins in the warm infusion and put compresses on the face. Change them 5-6 times. Leave each compress on the face for 5 minutes. A full course comprises 20-25 procedures. Apply half of them daily, and then every other day.

✔ Compresses with herbal infusion

- Calendula flowers
- Chamomile flowers
- Sage leaves
- Thyme
- Yarrow grass
- 200 ml of boiling water

Mix fresh herbs in equal parts: calendula flowers, chamomile flowers, sage leaves, thyme and yarrow grass. Add 2 tablespoons of this mixture to 200 ml of boiling water, leave to infuse for 30 minutes and filter. Use this infusion for compresses. A course comprises 20-25 procedures.

✔ Compress with cinquefoil extract

- 2 tablespoons of crushed cinquefoil rhizome

- 400 ml of water

Add 2 tablespoons of crushed cinquefoil rhizome to 200 ml of water, heat on a water bath for 30 minutes, stirring it slowly, then filter and let it cool down for 10 minutes. Use this extract for compresses to treat oily skin with acne.

Masks for acne skin care

✔ Mask with blue clay

- 1 tablespoon of blue clay

- 1-2 tablespoons of milk

Dissolve 1 tablespoon of blue clay in 1-2 tablespoons of milk and apply to the face for 15-20 minutes, then wash it off with warm water. Apply this mask before sleep once a week. A full course comprises 1-2 months. This is an effective remedy for acne.

✔ Yeast mask

- 40 g of fresh yeast

- Milk

Knead 40 g of fresh yeast with milk to the consistency of gruel and put on clean skin. Leave the mask for 20 minutes, then wash it off with warm water. This mask should be applied once a week.

✔ Mask with barley sprouts and peach

- 2 tablespoons of well-crushed barley sprouts

- 1 tablespoon of peach juice

- 3–5 drops of chamomile essential oil

Mix 2 tablespoons of well crushed barley sprouts with 1 tablespoon of peach juice. Add 3-5 drops of chamomile essential oil, stir and put the mask on your face for 20 minutes. Wash it off with cool water.

✔ Raspberry-milk mask

- 3 tablespoons of fresh raspberry juice

- 2 tablespoons of milk

Mix 3 tablespoons of fresh raspberry juice with 2 tablespoons of milk, moisten a napkin made from 2-3 layers of gauze in this mixture and apply to your face. Leave the mask for 15 minutes. Then wash it off with cool water.

✔ Cherry plum mask

- 6-7 ripe cherry plums

- 1 tablespoon of onion juice

- Half a tablespoon of olive oil

Knead 6-7 ripe cherry plums into pulp, add 1 tablespoon of onion juice and half a tablespoon of olive oil, stir thoroughly and apply this mixture to your face. Leave for 20 minutes, then wash it off with cool water.

✔ Quince mask

- 1 quince

Grate the quince on a plastic grater and apply the mass to your face. Leave the mask for 10-15 minutes. Then wash it off with cool water. If there is acne on your skin apply masks with quince daily or every other day. A full course comprises 15-20 procedures.

✓ Aloe mask

- Biostimulating aloe leaves

Wring the juice out of the biostimulating aloe leaves, moisten a gauze napkin folded in several layers in it, wring out slightly and apply to acne zones for 30-40 minutes. The full course of treatment comprises 30 procedures. Do the first 15 procedures daily, then every other day for 3 weeks and twice a week at the end of the course.

✓ Mask with chamomile

- 2 tablespoons of chamomile flowers
- 1 teaspoon of lemon juice
- 1 teaspoon of rye flour
- Boiling water

Add 2 tablespoons of chamomile flowers to a boiling water until you get a thick gruel, then add 1 teaspoon of lemon juice and 1 teaspoon of rye flour. Mix and apply this warm mask on skin with acne. Leave the mask for 20 minutes, then wash it off with cool water.

✓ Raspberry leaves mask

- Fresh raspberry leaves

Crush several fresh raspberry leaves, pound in a wooden mortar and apply to skin with acne for 15-20 minutes. Then wash it off with warm water. Raspberry leaves possess bactericidal properties and cleanse skin.

✔ Mask with plantain juice

- Plantain juice

Moisten a gauze napkin in fresh plantain juice and put it on your face, having applied a thin layer of cream first. Leave for 20 minutes. This mask is recommended for inflamed skin with acne.

✔ Mask with bur-marigold herb

- 4 tablespoons of crushed bur-marigold herb
- 200 ml of water

Add 4 tablespoons of crushed bur-marigold herb to 200 ml of water, heat on a water bath for 15 minutes, leave to infuse in a sealed vessel for 45 minutes and filter. Moisten a gauze napkin in this infusion and apply to the face. Leave the mask for 15 minutes. This procedure has anti-inflammatory and anti-allergic effects. Apply it twice a week.

✔ Mask with calendula

- 1 teaspoon of calendula tincture (40 g of calendula flowers, 200 ml of vodka)
- 100 ml of warm water

Dilute 1 teaspoon of calendula tincture (add 40 g of calendula flowers to 200 ml of vodka, leave to infuse for 2 weeks and filter) with 100 ml of warm water. Moisten a gauze napkin and put the mask on your face for 20 minutes. Such masks are useful for oily skin affected by seborrhea and acne. Carry out this procedure 2-3 times a week.

✔ Mask with tutsan extract

- Tutsan extract (1.5 tablespoons of tutsan herb, 200 ml of water)

Moisten a napkin in tutsan extract (1.5 tablespoons of herb per 200 ml of water) and apply the mask for 20 minutes, then apply a nourishing cream to your face. Carry out thie procedure daily for 10 days, then every other day. A full course comprises 25 procedures. These masks are recommended for effective acne treatment.

Compresses for facial skin with acne rosacea

If your facial skin is affected with acne rosacea it is best to apply cold compresses.

✓ Garlic compress

- 1 head of garlic
- 100 ml of vodka

Crush 1 head of garlic and add 100 ml of vodka. Leave to infuse for 2 hours and apply compress or wipe your face with this tincture once a day.

✓ Compress with aloe juice

- Aloe juice

Dilute aloe juice with water at a 1:2 ratio and apply the compress every other day. A full course comprises 20-25 procedures.

✓ Compress with bur-marigold herb extract

- 1.5 tablespoons of bur-marigold herb
- 200 ml of boiling water

Add 1.5 tablespoons of bur-marigold herb to 200 ml of boiling water, boil for10 minutes, let it cool down in a closed vessel and filter. Moisten a gauze napkin in this cold infusion and apply the lotion.

✔ **Compress with dill infusion**

- 2 teaspoons of dried dill seeds

- 100 ml of boiling water

Add 2 teaspoons of dried dill seeds to 100 ml of boiling water, leave to infuse for 1 hour and filter. Moisten a gauze napkin in this cold infusion and put compresses on affected skin zones. Leave for 20 minutes. Carry out this procedure for 2 weeks.

✔ **Compress with fireweed (Epilobium angustifolium) infusion**

- 3 tablespoons of fireweed leaves

- 200 ml of water

Add 3 tablespoons of fireweed leaves to 200 ml of water, heat on a water bath for 15 minutes, leave to infuse for 45 minutes and filter. Moisten a napkin in this infusion and apply compresses to your face daily. Leave the compress on your face for an hour, moistening the napkin in this infusion each 10-15 minutes. This compress is recommended for acne rosacea and psoriasis treatment.

Masks for facial skin with acne rosacea

Fruit and vegetable masks are best for acne rosacea. If you have oily skin, fruit, berry and vegetable juice may be mixed with egg white, and if your skin is dry and normal, with yolk or sour cream.

✔ **Tomato mask**

- 1 tablespoon of fresh tomato juice

- 1 tablespoon of sour cream or egg white

Mix 1 tablespoon of fresh tomato juice with 1 tablespoon of sour cream (for dry skin) or the egg white (for oily skin) and put this mixture on your face. Leave the mask for 10-15 minutes then wash it off. A full course comprises 20 procedures (every other day).

✔ Garlic mask

- Garlic

Pound garlic into gruel and apply it to your face once a week. Continue to carry out this procedure until full recovery.

✔ Cranberry mask

- Cranberries

Knead fresh cranberries in a wooden or porcelain mortar and wring out the juice. Moisten a gauze napkin in this juice and put the mask on your face, leave it for 10-15 minutes, then wash it off with water. This mask is recommended for oily skin with acne rosacea. A full course comprises 10-15 procedures. Apply masks daily until skin redness diminishes, then every other day and eventually twice a week. If the juice provokes skin irritation, you can dilute it with water at a 1:3 or 1:2 ratio.

✔ Ashberry mask

- 1 tablespoon of fresh juice of red ashberries

- 1 egg yolk

Mix 1 tablespoon of fresh juice of red ashberries with 1 egg yolk and put this mixture on the face. Leave the mask for 15 minutes. This is recommended for dry skin (if your skin is oily take an egg white instead of yolk). You can also apply masks with pure ashberry juice. Apply these masks twice a week. A full course comprises 15 procedures. If necessary (if skin irritation occurs) dilute the juice with water (1:1).

✔ Coriander mask

- 1 tablespoon of finely cut coriander greens
- 1 tablespoon of finely cut peppermint leaves
- Water

Add a small amount of water to 2 tablespoons of finely cut fresh coriander greens and peppermint leaves and stir to the consistency of gruel. Put the mask on your face for 15-20 minutes, then wash it off with soft warm water. If you have dry skin prone to redness and irritation, you may spread your face with softening lotion after this procedure.

✔ Dill mask

- Fresh dill
- 1 egg white

Crush fresh dill and mix with 1 egg white in equal parts. Apply this mask every other day, leave for 20 minutes, then wash it off with warm water. Carry out this procedure for a month.

✔ Melissa mask

- 40 g of melissa
- 200 ml of vodka
- 1 tablespoon of sour cream
- 1 teaspoon of vegetable oil
- 1 g of baker's yeast
- Oatmeal

To prepare the melissa tincture add 40 g of herb to 200 ml of vodka, leave to infuse for a week and filter. Mix 1 tablespoon of melissa tincture with 1 tablespoon of sour cream, 1 teaspoon of vegetable oil and 1 g of baker's yeast. Add oatmeal and stir everything thoroughly to the consistency of a thick cream. Put this mixture on the face and leave the mask for 10-15 minutes. Wash it off with warm water, then with cool water. Apply this mask twice a week for 2 months. This mask eliminates skin itching and bleaches freckles and pigment spots.

✔ Parsley mask

- 2 tablespoons of crushed parsley greens and roots

- 1 egg white

Mix 2 tablespoons of crushed parsley greens and roots with the egg white and apply to your face daily. Leave the mask for 15 minutes. A full course comprises 15 procedures.

Tinctures, infusions and decoctions for bleaching facial skin with pigment spots and freckles

✔ Parsley tincture with lemon juice

- 50 g of finely cut parsley greens

- Half a liter of vodka

- 2 tablespoons of lemon juice

Add 50 g of finely cut parsley greens to half a liter of vodka, add 2 tablespoons of lemon juice and leave to infuse in a dark place for 2 weeks. Then filter and use for facial skin with bleaching freckles and pigment spots.

✔ Parsley infusion

- 1 glass of finely cut parsley greens

- 200 ml of boiling water

Add 1 glass of finely cut parsley greens to 200 ml of boiling water. Leave to infuse for 30 minutes and filter. Wipe your face with this infusion 2-3 times a day. You can apply parsley juice to bleach skin as well.

✔ Parsley and chamomile infusion

- 2 tablespoons of fresh parsley

- 2 tablespoons of chamomile flowers

- Half a liter of water

Add 4 tablespoons of fresh parsley and chamomile flowers to half a liter of water and let it infuse for a day. Wipe facial skin with freckles with this infusion several times a day. This is an effective remedy for freckle discoloration.

✔ Dandelion infusion

- 1 tablespoon of fresh dandelion flowers

- 200 ml of water

Add 1 tablespoon of fresh dandelion flowers to 200 ml of water, heat on a water bath for 10-15 minutes, let it infuse for 45 minutes and filter. Wipe freckles and pigment spots with this infusion in the morning and in the evening. You can also wipe skin with fresh dandelion juice, then after it dries wipe the face with whey or curdled milk.

✔ Elecampane decoction

- 1 tablespoon of crushed elecampane roots

- 200 ml of water

Add 1 tablespoon of crushed elecampane roots to 200 ml of water, heat on a water bath for 30 minutes and let it cool down for10 minutes. Filter this decoction and wipe freckles with it once or twice a day.

Lotions for facial skin with pigment spots and freckles

✔ Rice lotion

- 2 tablespoons of rice

- 300 ml of cool water

- 2 tablespoons of lemon or cranberry juice

Add 2 tablespoons of rice to 300 ml of cool water and leave to infuse for 2 hours. Then filter this infusion and add 2 tablespoons of lemon or cranberry juice. Stir well and wipe facial skin with freckles and pigment spots with this lotion daily before sleep for two weeks.

✔ Cucumber lotion

- 1 cucumber

- 2 tablespoons of olive oil

Grate the cucumber on a plastic grater and wring out the juice. Mix 2 tablespoons of cucumber juice with 2 tablespoons of olive oil. Wipe facial skin with this lotion to bleach freckles and pigment spots.

✔ Lemon lotion

- 50 ml of lemon juice

- 250 ml of light rum

- 1 teaspoon of glycerin

Add 250 ml of light rum and 1 teaspoon of glycerin to 50 ml of lemon juice. This lotion bleaches skin.

✔ Lotion with calendula and lemon juice

- 2 tablespoons of fresh calendula petal juice

- 2 tablespoons of lemon juice

Mix 2 tablespoons of fresh calendula petal juice with 2 tablespoons of lemon juice and wipe freckles and pigment spots with the lotion.

✔ **Egg-lemon lotion**

- 1 egg white

- 2 tablespoons of lemon juice

- 1 teaspoon of glycerin

- 100 ml of vodka

Whip the egg white carefully and mix with 2 tablespoons of lemon juice. Add 1 teaspoon of glycerin and 100 ml of vodka. Wipe your skin with this lotion in the evening.

✔ **Ashberry-lemon lotion**

- 2 tablespoons of red ashberry juice

- 2 tablespoons of lemon juice

- 2 tablespoons of parsley juice

- 40 ml of vodka

Mix 2 tablespoons of red ashberry juice, lemon juice and parsley juice and add 40 ml of vodka. Wipe your face with this lotion to discolor freckles and pigment spots.

✔ **Lotion with parsley 1**

- 1 tablespoon of parsley juice

- 1 tablespoon of milk

Mix 1 tablespoon of fresh parsley juice with 1 tablespoon of milk and wipe your face once a day. Wash the lotion off with cool water after 15 minutes.

✔ **Lotion with parsley 2**

- 1 tablespoon of crushed parsley greens

- 100 ml of boiling water

- 1 tablespoon of viburnum juice

- Half a tablespoon of lemon juice

Add 1 tablespoon of crushed parsley greens to 100 ml of boiling water and leave to infuse in a tightly sealed vessel for 30 minutes. Then filter and add 1 tablespoon of viburnum juice and half a tablespoon of lemon juice. Wipe freckles and pigment spots with this lotion daily before sleep. Carry out this procedure for two weeks.

Bleaching masks for facial skin with pigment spots and freckles

It is important to apply bleaching masks in the evening so as to avoid exposure to the sun.

✓ Sour-milk mask

- 50 ml of curdled milk or yoghurt

- 1 tablespoon of oat flakes

Mix 50 ml of curdled milk or yoghurt with 1 tablespoon of oat flakes to the consistency of gruel. Put this mixture on a linen napkin and cover your face with it. Leave the mask for 10-15 minutes. Then wash it off with cool water. It is recommended for bleaching of freckles and pigment spots, especially for oily skin.

✓ Mustard mask

- Mustard powder

- Warm water

Dissolve the mustard powder in the warm water and mix to the consistency of gruel. Wipe pigment spots every other day. As soon as you feel burning, wash the mask off. A course comprises

10 procedures. It is not recommended that you apply this mask if you have varicose blood vessels or hypertrichosis.

✓ Mask with oat bran

- Oat bran

- Hot milk

Mix the oat bran with hot milk to the consistency of gruel and put this mixture on the face. Leave the mask for 10-15 minutes. Then wash it off with warm water.

✓ Oat mask with sauerkraut juice

- 2 tablespoons of oatmeal

- 2 tablespoons of sauerkraut juice

Mix 2 tablespoons of oatmeal with 2 tablespoons of sauerkraut juice, put this mixture on your face for 15 minutes, then wash it off. This mask is recommended for bleaching of freckles and pigment spots.

✓ Almond mask

- Half a glass of peeled almonds

- 200 ml of boiling water

- 1 tablespoon of lemon juice

- 1 teaspoon of honey

Add half a glass of peeled almonds to 200 ml of boiling water and leave for 10 minutes, then pour the almond water into a separate pan and mince the almonds in a mincing machine. Add 1 tablespoon of lemon juice and 1 teaspoon of honey. Stir and dilute with water to the consistency of gruel. Put the mask on your face, leave for 20 minutes, then wash it off with almond water. Apply this mask in case of moderate pigmentation, it possesses soft bleaching properties.

✓ Pumpkin seeds mask 1

- Peeled raw pumpkin seeds

- 1 tablespoon of water

- 1 tablespoon of honey

Knead 1 tablespoon of peeled raw pumpkin seeds carefully in a wooden or porcelain mortar with 1 tablespoon of water. Add 1 tablespoon of honey to the pumpkin milk, stir well and put the mask on your face. Leave for 20 minutes, then wash it off with warm water. Carry out this procedure every day until freckles and pigment spots become colorless.

✓ Pumpkin seeds mask 2

- Pumpkin seeds

- Olive oil

To bleach freckles mix pounded pumpkin seeds with olive oil to the consistency of gruel and put this mask on your skin every day.

✓ Haricot mask

- 50 g of boiled haricot

- 3 teaspoons of sunflower or olive oil

Knead 50 g of boiled haricot, add 3 teaspoons of sunflower or olive oil and put this mixture on your face. Leave for 20 minutes, then wash it off with water. This mask helps to discolor freckles and pigment spots.

✓ Cucumber mask 1

- 1 cucumber

Put fresh cucumber juice on freckles and pigment spots in several layers and leave for 40-50 minutes each day for 20 days.

Then wash the mask off and spread your skin with a nourishing cream.

✔ Cucumber mask 2

- 2 tablespoons of fresh cucumber

- 2 tablespoons of vodka

Mix 2 tablespoons of fresh cucumber, grated on a small plastic grater, with 2 tablespoons of vodka and leave to infuse for four hours. Then filter, moisten a gauze or linen napkin in this infusion and put the mask on your face. Leave for 15 minutes, then wash it off with cool water. Carry out this procedure for a month.

✔ Horseradish mask 1

- 2 tablespoons of grated horseradish

- 1 apple, pulped

Mix 2 tablespoons of grated horseradish and fresh apple pulp. Put the mask on your face, leave for 20 minutes, then wash it off with cool water. This mask bleaches skin well.

✔ Horseradish mask 2

- 50 ml of curdled milk

- 1 teaspoon of grated horseradish

- 1 tablespoon of oatmeal

Mix 50 ml of curdled milk with 1 teaspoon of grated horseradish, add 1 tablespoon of oatmeal and stir well. Put the mask on your face for 20 minutes. Then wash it off with cool water. This mask bleaches skin effectively.

✔ Horseradish mask 3

- 1 teaspoon of grated horseradish

- 1 tablespoon of sour cream

- 1 tablespoon of lemon juice

Mix 2 tablespoons of grated horseradish, sour cream and lemon juice. Put this mixture on the face, leave for 10-15 minutes and wash it off with warm water at first, then with cold water. The mask bleaches skin effectively.

✔ Yeast mask with lemon

- 20 g of yeast

- 2 teaspoons of lemon pulp

Mix 20 g of yeast with 2 teaspoons of mashed pulp of a lemon. Warm this mixture a little on a water bath and put on your face until it is warm. Leave the mask for 20-30 minutes and wash it off with warm water. This bleaching mask is suitable for all types of skin.

✔ Lemon mask

- Lemon juice

Lemon juice discolors freckles and pigment spots. It is useful to put several layers of it on the face daily. Wash it off in 40-50 minutes and spread your skin with a nourishing cream. Carry out this procedure for 20 days.

✔ Lemon-honey mask with parsley

- 1 tablespoon of lemon juice

- 1 tablespoon of honey

- 1 tablespoon of crushed parsley greens

Mix 2 tablespoons of lemon juice and honey, add 1 tablespoon of crushed parsley greens. Put this mixture on the facial skin and leave the mask for 15 minutes. Wash it off with cool water.

✔ Lemon mask with starch

- Lemon juice

- Starch

Mix the lemon juice and starch in equal parts and put this mixture on your skin. Leave the mask for 15 minutes. Then wash it off with cool water.

✔ Lemon juice and cream mask

- 1 teaspoon of cream

- 1 teaspoon of lemon juice

Mix 1 teaspoon of cream with1 teaspoon of lemon juice. Put this mask on your face with a cotton wool ball, leave for 20 minutes, then wash it off. This mask bleaches and rejuvenates skin well.

✔ Lemon- currant mask

- 1 teaspoon of lemon juice

- Red currants

- Dandelion flowers

- 1 teaspoon of olive or sunflower-seed oil

Mix 1 teaspoon of lemon juice, kneaded red currants and crushed dandelion flowers with1 teaspoon of olive or sunflower-seed oil. Put this mask on problem zones of your skin for 20 minutes. Wash it off with cool water. Carry out this procedure in the morning and in the evening.

✔ Lemon-carrot mask

- 2 tablespoons of fresh carrot juice

- 1 teaspoon of lemon juice

Mix 2 tablespoons of fresh carrot juice with 1 teaspoon of lemon juice and spread your skin with it. In 30 minutes wash it off. Carry out this procedure 2-3 times a day.

✔ Pineapple mask

- Pineapple

- 1 tablespoon of sour cream or natural yoghurt

- 1 teaspoon of honey

Mix 1 tablespoon of mashed pulp of the pineapple with1 tablespoon of sour cream or natural yoghurt and 1 teaspoon of honey. Put this mixture on skin for 20 minutes. Then wash it off with warm water. Pineapple lightens freckles, bleaches skin slightly and makes it elastic.

✔ Berry mask

- Vegetable oil

- Cranberries, red currants, gooseberries or wild strawberries

Knead cranberries, red currants, gooseberries or wild strawberries and put on your face (having greased it with vegetable oil first). Leave the mask for 10-15 minutes. Then wash it off with cool water. Apply this bleaching mask 2-3 times a week. A course comprises15-20 procedures. You can also wipe freckles with the juice of these berries once or twice a day.

✔ Gooseberries mask

- 1 tablespoon of kneaded unripe gooseberries

- 1 tablespoon of sour cream

Mix 1 tablespoon of kneaded unripe gooseberries with1 tablespoon of sour cream and apply the mask to your face. Leave for 20 minutes, then wash it off with warm water. This mask is useful for flabby skin and for discoloration of freckles.

✔ Raspberry mask

- Overripe raspberries

Knead overripe raspberries and put this gruel on your face. Leave the mask for 15 minutes. Then wash it off with cool water. This mask clears and moistens skin well, bleaches freckles.

✔ Strawberry mask

- Fresh wild strawberry juice

Put the juice of fresh wild strawberries on your face. Leave the mask for 10-15 minutes, then wash it off with cool water. You can also wipe freckles and pigment spots with this juice daily. Juice of fresh wild strawberries is an ancient cosmetic means for their discoloration.

✔ Viburnum juice mask

- Viburnum juice

Moisten a gauze or linen napkin in fresh viburnum juice and put the mask on your face. Leave for 20-30 minutes. Viburnum juice bleaches freckles and pigment spots well.

✔ Melissa mask

- 1 tablespoon of melissa
- 200 ml of water

Masks with melissa infusion (1 tablespoon of herb per 200 ml of water) are recommended for skin with pigment spots.

✔ Dandelion mask 1

- 8–10 fresh dandelion leaves
- 1 tablespoon of low-fat curds

- Whey or yoghurt

Crush 8-10 fresh dandelion leaves carefully and mix with 1 tablespoon of low-fat curds. Put the mask on your face, having spread spots and freckles with the dandelion juice first. In 15-20 minutes remove the mask with a cotton wool ball and wipe your skin with whey or yoghurt.

✔ Dandelion mask 2

- 2 tablespoons of fresh dandelion flowers

Knead 2 tablespoons of fresh dandelion flowers until juice appears. Put this mask on the face and leave for 20 minutes, then wash it off with cool water. This mask bleaches skin and makes it healthy.

✔ Dandelion mask 3

- 1 tablespoon of dandelion juice

- 1 tablespoon of parsley juice

Mix 2 tablespoons of dandelion and parsley juice. Apply this mixture to your face and wash it off in 15 minutes.

Bleaching creams for facial skin with pigment spots and freckles

Take care not to spread your face with bleaching creams before going out.

✔ Cucumber cream 1

- 1 fresh cucumber

- 30 g of nourishing cream

If you have dry skin grate a cucumber on a small plastic grater, add 30 g of any nourishing cream for dry skin and apply to your face.

✓ Cucumber cream 2

- 1 fresh cucumber

- 15 g of lanolin

- 50 ml of sesame oil

Grate the cucumber on a plastic grater. Then melt 15 g of lanolin on a water bath, add 50 ml of sesame oil and 1 tablespoon of the cucumber paste. Leave this mixture on a water bath for an hour, then filter, stir well and let it cool down.

✓ Cream with white lily

- 10 g of beeswax

- 1 teaspoon of honey

- 3 tablespoons of crushed petals of white lily

- 2 teaspoons of garlic juice

Melt 10 g of beeswax on a water bath and add 2 teaspoons of honey, 3 tablespoons of crushed white lily petals and 2 teaspoons of garlic juice. Stir well, take off the water bath and let it cool down. This cream not only bleaches skin, but also prevents the occurrence of wrinkles.

Sunburn protection

✓ Lemon water

- 1 lemon

- 1 glass of cold water

Add several slices of lemon to a glass of cold water and leave to infuse for one night. Use this water to protect your skin against solar burns.

✔ Tea brew

- 1 teaspoon of tea
- 50 ml of boiling water

To prevent solar burns wipe your skin with strong cold tea before going out (1 teaspoon of tea per 50 ml of boiling water).

✔ Oil cream with tea

- 2 tablespoons of lanolin
- Half a tablespoon of almond oil
- 1 tablespoon of sesame oil
- 1 teaspoon of tea
- 50 ml of boiling water
- 4-5 drops of lavender or chamomile essential oil

Melt 2 tablespoons of lanolin on a water bath, add half a tablespoon of almond oil and 1 tablespoon of sesame oil and then, stirring constantly, add 50 ml of strong tea brew (1 teaspoon of tea per 50 ml of boiling water). Let it cool down, add 4-5 drops of lavender or chamomile essential oil and stir well. This cream moistens skin and protects it from ultraviolet rays.

✔ Sesame oil

- Sesame oil

Sesame oil is a perfect natural means, possessing sun protection properties.

✔ Olive and coconut oils

- Olive and coconut oils

These oils absorb ultraviolet rays. You can use them while sunbathing.

Compresses on sunburns

✔ Tutsan extract

- 1 tablespoon of tutsan herb

- 200 ml of water

Add 1 tablespoon of tutsan herb to 200 ml of water, heat on a water bath for 30 minutes, filter and let it cool down for 10 minutes. Moisten your sunburnt skin with this extract or apply a compress.

✔ Peppermint infusion

- 1 tablespoon of peppermint leaves

- 200 ml of boiling water

Add 1 tablespoon of peppermint leaves to 200 ml of boiling water, leave to infuse in a closed vessel for 30 minutes and filter. Moisten your sunburnt skin with this infusion and apply compress.

✔ Compress with haricot infusion

- Handful of haricot flowers

- 250 ml of boiling water

Add a handful of haricot flowers to 250 ml of boiling water and leave to infuse in a sealed vessel for an hour. Cool in a refrigerator without filtering, then moisten a gauze napkin in this infusion and put it on your face. Leave the compress for 30 minutes.

✔ Compress with mountain arnica tincture

- 20 g of mountain arnica flowers
- 200 ml of vodka

Moisten a gauze napkin in mountain arnica tincture (add 20 g of mountain arnica flowers to 200 ml of vodka, leave to infuse for 7-10 days and filter), diluted with water at a 1:1 ratio and apply to sunburnt skin.

✔ Compress with oak extract

- 40 g of crushed oak bark
- 400 ml of water

Add 40 g of crushed oak bark to 200 ml of water, heat on a water bath for 30 minutes, filter and cool it. Apply cold lotions with this extract for one hour, changing them five to six times.

✔ Compress with chamomile infusion

- 1 tablespoon of chamomile flowers
- 200 ml of boiling water

Add 1 tablespoon of chamomile flowers to 200 ml of boiling water, leave to infuse for one hour, filter and apply compresses on solar burns.

✔ Compress with nettle infusion

- 2 tablespoons of crushed nettle leaves
- 200 ml of boiling water

Add 2 tablespoons of crushed nettle leaves to 200 ml of boiling water, leave to infuse for one hour and filter. Use this infusion for compresses on solar burns.

✓ Cucumber juice

- Cucumber juice

Moisten sunburnt areas with cucumber juice or apply slices of a fresh cucumber for 15-20 minutes.

✓ Watermelon juice

- Watermelon juice

Moisten your sunburnt skin with watermelon juice.

Masks on sunburns

✓ Yoghurt mask

- Yoghurt or kefir

Put yoghurt or kefir on your skin and after 20 minutes wash it off with some water.

✓ Egg-curd mask

- 1 tablespoon of curds

- 1 tablespoon of sour cream

- 1 egg white

Knead 1 tablespoon of curds with 1 tablespoon of sour cream and mix with the whipped egg white. Put this mixture on your sunburnt skin for 15-20 minutes, then wash it off.

✓ Yolk mask

- 1 egg yolk

Apply raw egg yolk on your sunburnt skin. Leave the mask for 10-15 minutes, then wash it off with water.

✔ Potato mask

- Raw potato

- Oat or wheat flour

Wring the juice out of a grated raw potato, add a little oat or wheat flour, stir to the consistency of liquid gruel and apply it to sunburnt skin. Leave the mask for 15 minutes. You can also apply warm mashed potatoes mask mixed with cream or sour cream.

✔ Starch mask

- Starch

- Cold water

In case of solar burns mix starch with cold water to the consistency of gruel, apply it to your skin with a cotton wool ball and let it dry. Then wash it off with boiled water. This mask removes redness and skin inflammation.

✔ Strawberry mask

- Strawberries

- 1 tablespoon of milk

Mix several pounded strawberries with1 tablespoon of milk. Apply this mixture to sunburnt skin and leave for 15-20 minutes.

✔ Apricot mask

- 1 apricot

Apply apricot pulp to sunburnt areas of your skin and leave for 15-20 minutes.

✔ Banana mask

- Half a ripe banana

- 1 teaspoon of honey

- Half a tablespoon of oatmeal

Knead half of a ripe banana, add1 teaspoon of honey and half a tablespoon of oatmeal. Stir well. Apply this mixture to sunburnt skin for 15-20 minutes, then wash it off with water. This mask moistens and calms skin, removing burning and redness.

✔ Mask with salad

- Salad leaves

- Water

Add salad leaves to a small amount of water and boil for 5 minutes. Filter the broth, chop some salad leaves, put them on a gauze napkin and cover your face with this mask. Leave it for 20-25 minutes, then wash it off with the salad broth. Carry out this procedure several times a day. It calms sunburnt skin, removing redness. Wipe your face with the salad broth as well.

✔ Oil for sunburnt skin 1

- Dandelion roots

- Wheat sprout oil

Mix crushed dandelion roots with wheat sprout oil (at a 1:10 ratio) and leave to infuse for one day. Then heat this mixture on a water bath for 1 hour and filter. Spread burnt areas of your skin with this oil several times a day. Store this oil in a dark place.

✔ Oil for sunburnt skin 2

- Lavender essential oil

If your skin is badly burnt you should apply lavender essential oil.

Skin care recipes for the skin around the eyes

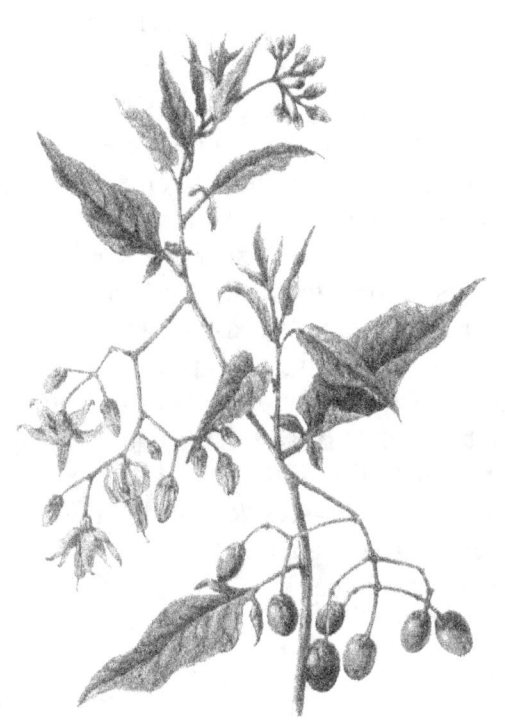

Caring for skin around the eyes

Skin around the eyes is gentle and thin and should be treated with care. There are no sebaceous glands present, and wrinkles appear here very early. It is thus important that you start taking care of the skin around your eyes as soon as possible. Dark circles and bags under the eyes are characteristics of tired skin. They appear due to stresses, sleeplessness, nervous fatigue, bright sunlight, bad meals and long working conditions with insufficient illumination (or with excessively bright light sources).

Edematous eyelids present a great problem for those who are over 30. The main reason for that is liquid retention. Moisturizing and blood circulation within the skin worsen; the skin becomes thinner, transparent, and it is most visible on the eyelids. Dark circles and edemas under eyes can testify to liver and kidney diseases or hypertension. However, if the symptoms are not connected with internal diseases, you can get rid of them rather easily. Biologically active substances contained in medicinal plants such as parsley, sage, horsetail, etc. can help, as they strengthen the outflow of lymphatic liquid. Cold compresses stimulating blood circulation are also useful. After lotions, eye baths and compresses you need to apply a thin layer of nourishing cream. Do so cautiously with your finger tips, making sure not to stretch the skin.

Anti-wrinkle recipes for skin around the eyes

✔ **Oil massage**

- Almond or olive oil

To prevent the occurrence of wrinkles in the corners of the eyes, apply an oil massage. Every day put almond or olive oil on the eyelids and skin round the eyes and tap it with slight finger movements. You can also add several drops of rose or sandalwood essential oil.

✓ **Compresses with birch infusion**

- Fresh birch leaves

- Water

Fill a glass with fresh birch leaves, pour cold water over the top and leave to infuse for 8 hours. Moisten cotton wool balls in this infusion and apply to the skin around the eyes. Leave compresses for 10-15 minutes, then apply a thin layer of a nourishing cream.

✓ **Yolk-honey mask**

- 1 egg yolk

- Half a tablespoon of honey

- 50 ml of vegetable oil

At the occurrence of wrinkles around the eyes, apply a softening mask: knead the egg yolk with 2.5 tablespoons of honey and 50 ml of vegetable oil until you get a consistent texture. Apply this mixture to the skin around the eyes (and if you have dry irritable skin, to the whole face) for 15-20 minutes. Then wash it off first with warm water, and then with cool.

✓ **Oil mask**

- 2 teaspoons of sea-buckthorn oil

- 2 teaspoons of cocoa oil

- 5-8 drops of vitamin E oil solution

To help battle wrinkles in the corners of the eyes mix 2 teaspoons of sea-buckthorn oil and cocoa oil rendered on a water bath and add 5-8 drops of vitamin E oil solution. Put a thick layer of this mixture on the eyelids and the areas with wrinkles. After 15 minutes remove the mask and dry skin with a napkin. This mask effectively smoothes wrinkles. This mask should be applied three times a week in the evening before sleep.

✔ Potato mask

- 1 potato
- 1 teaspoon of sour cream
- Cold tea

This mask is recommended for flabby skin under the eyes covered with small wrinkles. Boil the potato in its skin, peel it and mix with 1 teaspoon of sour cream. Put this warm mixture on the skin under your eyes, beginning from the external corners of the eyes. Leave the mask for 15-20 minutes, then remove it and apply some cream to the eyelids with easy movements, from external corners to internal. In 10-15 minutes remove the remains of the cream with a cotton wool ball moistened in cold tea.

✔ Vitamin cream

- 1 teaspoon of cream
- 1 drop of vitamin A oil solution
- 1 drop of vitamin E oil solution

Add 1 drop of vitamins A and E to 1 teaspoon of fresh cream. This cream is effective against wrinkles in the corners of the eyes, improving complexion and making skin fresh and healthy.

✔ Almond cream

- 1 tablespoon of lanolin
- 2 tablespoons of almond oil
- 1 teaspoon of lecithin
- 2 tablespoons of cool water

Melt 1 tablespoon of lanolin on a water bath and add 2 tablespoons of almond oil. Take the mixture off the water bath and, stirring constantly, add 1 teaspoon of lecithin and 2 tablespoons of cool water little-by-little. Use the prepared cream for caring for skin around the eyes.

Compresses for dark circles around the eyes

✓ Curd compress

- 2 teaspoons of curds

Wrap 2 teaspoons of curds in 2 gauze napkins and put them on your eyes for 10 minutes. After this compress apply some nourishing cream to the skin around the eyes.

✓ Oil compress

- Olive oil

Moisten cotton wool balls in warm olive oil, apply to the skin under your eyes and leave while the compress remains warm. Repeat this procedure every day; if necessary, for several weeks.

✓ Potato compress

- Raw potatoes

Grate the potatoes on a plastic grater, wring out the juice, moisten cotton wool balls in it and apply to the skin under your eyes for 15-20 minutes. After this compress apply a thin layer of nourishing cream.

✓ Tea compress

- 1 teaspoon of tea

- 50 ml of boiling water

Moisten cotton wool balls in cold tea brew and apply to your eyes for 10 minutes. Change compresses several times. After the compress apply some nourishing cream on wet skin.

You can also use tea bags as compresses. Dip them into boiling water for a few seconds, let them cool down and apply to your eyes.

✔ Compress with parsley

- Fresh parsley root

Peel the parsley root, mince and apply the gruel to the skin under your eyes. Leave the compress for 15-20 minutes, then wash it off with warm water. This compress is very useful in the case of dark circles under your eyes and edematous eyelids.

✔ Compress with dill

- 1 teaspoon of dill greens
- 100 ml of boiling water

Add 1 teaspoon of dill greens to 100 ml of boiling water and leave to infuse for 10-15 minutes. Moisten cotton wool balls in this infusion and apply to the skin under your eyes. You can also fill small gauze bags with dill seeds, dip them into boiling water for 15 minutes, cool them a little and use as compresses (procedure time: 10 minutes).

Compresses and masks for edemas under the eyes

✔ Compress with cucumber juice

- 1 fresh cucumber
- Rose water

Grate a fresh cucumber on a plastic grater, wring out the juice and put it in a refrigerator. Then moisten two gauze napkins in rose water at first, and then in cold cucumber juice and apply to your eyes twice a day. This compress freshens skin round the eyes. After this compress apply a thin layer of nourishing cream.

✔ Mint compress

- 1 tablespoon of peppermint leaves
- 250 ml of boiling water

In case of edemas under your eyes and edematous eyelids add 1 tablespoon of peppermint leaves to 250 ml of boiling water, boil on a low heat for 5 minutes and let it infuse in a sealed vessel for 30 minutes. Then filter the infusion, moisten cotton wool balls in it and apply them to your eyes for 10-15 minutes. After this procedure apply a nourishing cream to the skin around the eyes.

✔ Contrast compresses with sage or chamomile

- 1 tablespoon of sage leaves or chamomile flowers

- 200 ml of boiled water

Add 1 tablespoon of sage leaves or chamomile flowers to 200 ml of boiled water, heat on a water bath for 15 minutes, then leave to infuse in a sealed vessel for 45 minutes and filter. Cool one half of the infusion in a refrigerator and warm the other half. Then moisten cotton wool balls in cold and warm infusions in turns and apply to your eyes. Leave the warm compresses for 20-30 seconds and the cold compresses for 3-5 seconds. Repeat this procedure 5-6 times, finishing with cold compress. Then put some nourishing cream on the eyelids and skin under your eyes. Carry out this procedure every other day.

✔ Compress with parsley infusion

- 1 tablespoon of crushed parsley greens

- 200 ml of boiling water

Add 1 tablespoon of crushed parsley greens to 200 ml of boiling water, leave to infuse for 15-20 minutes and filter. Moisten cotton wool balls in the warm infusion and put them on the eyelids and skin under your eyes for 10 minutes every morning and every evening for a month.

✔ Compress with chamomile infusion

- 1 tablespoon of chamomile flowers

- 200 ml of boiled water

Add 1 tablespoon of chamomile flowers to 200 ml of boiled water, heat on a water bath for 15 minutes, leave to infuse for 45 minutes and filter. Moisten cotton wool balls in this infusion and put them on your eyes.

✔ **Compress with horsetail extract**

- 1 tablespoon of field horsetail herb

- 250 ml of water

Add 1 tablespoon of field horsetail herb to 250 ml of water, heat on a water bath for 30 minutes, then cool at room temperature for 10 minutes and filter. Moisten cotton wool balls in the cold extract and put them on your eyes for 10-15 minutes. These compresses remove edemas and help with eye exhaustion.

✔ **Ice compress**

- Cubes of ice with herbal infusions

Place ice cubes into polyethylene bags and put on edemas under your eyes for 5 minutes. You can use herbal infusions (chamomile, parsley, mint, etc.) to prepare the ice or brew tea bags in boiling water and then freeze them in a refrigerator and put on your eyelids. This compress quickly removes edemas under eyes.

✔ **Potato mask 1**

- 1 raw potato

Put thin slices of raw potato around the eyes and on eyelids for 10-15 minutes . This mask helps with exhaustion, inflammation and edemas, freshening the skin around the eyes.

✔ **Potato mask 2**

- 1 raw potato

Grate the potato on a small plastic grater and apply the potato paste to the skin under your eyes for 10-15 minutes. Then remove the mask with a cotton wool balls moistened in cold tea and apply some nourishing cream.

✓ Potato mask 3

- 1 small potato
- Parsley greens

Mix one small grated potato with crushed parsley greens. Wrap this mixture in gauze napkins and place on your eyelids and edemas under your eyes for 10-15 minutes. Then apply a nourishing cream.

✓ Milk-potato mask

- 1 teaspoon of grated raw potato
- 1 teaspoon of wheat flour
- 1 teaspoon of milk

Mix 1 teaspoon of grated raw potato and wheat flour, add 1 teaspoon of milk and stir thoroughly. Put this mixture on gauze napkins and cover the skin under your eyes with this mask for 10-15 minutes. Remove it with a cotton wool ball moistened in cold tea brew.

✓ Cucumber mask

- 1 fresh cucumber

This is a true and tried folk remedy for edematous eyelids, that tones skin well. Put slices of a fresh cucumber on your eyelids and skin round the eyes. Leave the mask for 10-15 minutes.

✓ Parsley mask

- Parsley greens

Crush fresh parsley greens carefully and put on your eyelids and skin under the eyes. Then cover them with cotton wool balls moistened in cool water. Leave the mask for 15 minutes.

Compresses, baths and masks for eye irritation, inflammation and edematous eyelids

✔ Milk compress

- Warm milk

In case of reddened eyes and eyelids moisten two cotton wool balls with warm milk and put on your eyelids for 10-15 minutes.

✔ Compress with rose water

- Rose water

In case of hematopsia moisten two cotton wool balls in rose water and put on your eyelids. Leave for 20-30 minutes. This compress also relieves eye exhaustion, bringing back a healthy shine.

✔ Compress with bluebottle infusion

- Half a tablespoon of bluebottle flowers
- 200 ml of water

The bluebottle infusion removes irritation and allergic reaction, promoting skin regeneration. Add half a tablespoon of bluebottle marginal flowers to 200 ml of water, heat in a closed vessel on a water bath for 15 minutes, cool at room temperature for 45 minutes and filter. Put cotton wool ball or gauze napkins moistened in this infusion on your eyes for 10-15 minutes.

✔ Compress with birch extract

- 1 tablespoon of birch buds or leaves

- 250 ml of boiling water

Add 1 tablespoon of birch buds or leaves to 250 ml of boiling water, boil on a low heat for 10-15 minutes, let it cool down at room temperature and filter. Make compresses with this extract for exhausted and inflamed eyes.

✔ **Baths with eyebright or fennel herbs**

- 3 teaspoons of eyebright or fennel herbs

- 400 ml of boiling water

Add 3 teaspoons of eyebright or fennel herbs to 400 ml of boiling water, leave to infuse for 20-30 minutes and filter. Pour this infusion, cooled to room temperature, into an eye bath. Wash your eyes in turns for 30 seconds.

✔ **Mint compress**

- 1 tablespoon of peppermint leaves

- 250 ml of water

Mint compresses are recommended for edematous eyelids. Add 1 tablespoon of peppermint leaves to 250 ml of water, heat on a water bath for 15 minutes, leave to infuse for 45 minutes and filter. Moisten cotton wool balls in the mint infusion and put on your eyelids for 10 minutes.

✔ **Potato compress with fennel**

- 2 tablespoons of crushed raw potato, grated

- 2 tablespoons of crushed fresh fennel

Mix 2 tablespoons of crushed fresh fennel and grated raw potato. Wrap this paste in two gauze napkins and put on your eyes for 10 minutes. This compress effectively relieves eye exhaustion.

✔ Compress with chamomile flowers

- Chamomile flowers
- Boiling water

In case of severe eye inflammation and swollen eyelids fill small linen sacks with chamomile flowers and dip them in boiling water for 5-10 minutes. Let them cool down a little and put the warm bags on your eyes. This compress has a calming effect and removes irritation. With regular application 2-3 times a week it also prevents the occurrence of wrinkles around the eyes.

If you have inflamed reddened eyes, you can also apply lotions with chamomile tincture, putting a napkin moistened in this infusion on your eyes for 3-5 minutes.

✔ Compress with birch infusion

- 1 tablespoon of birch leaves
- 200 ml of water

In case of edematous eyelids add1 tablespoon of birch leaves to 200 ml of water, leave to infuse for 8 hours and filter. Then moisten cotton wool balls with this infusion and put them on your eyelids for 10-15 minutes.

✔ Compress with eyebright infusion

- 1 tablespoon of eyebright herb
- 200 ml of water

This compress is very effective against eyelid inflammation and tear-bags. Add 1 tablespoon of eyebright herb to 200 ml of water, heat on a water bath for 15 minutes, leave to infuse for 45 minutes and filter. Moisten cotton wool balls in this infusion and apply them in turns for 10-15 minutes.

✔ Compress with linden infusion

- 1 tablespoon of linden flowers

- 200 ml of boiling water

In case of eye exhaustion and edematous eyelids add 1 tablespoon of linden flowers to 200 ml of boiling water, leave to infuse in a sealed vessel for 30 minutes and filter. Moisten a gauze napkin in this infusion, wring it out slightly and put on your eyes for 3-5 minutes. This infusion also smoothes small wrinkles around the eyes. Washing the eyes with linden infusion is also an option for reddened eyelids.

✔ Compress with parsley infusion

- 1 tablespoon of crushed parsley greens

- 200 ml of boiling water

Compresses and rinsing with parsley infusion are useful for irritation and dim eye coloration. Add 1 tablespoon of crushed parsley greens to 200 ml of boiling water, leave to infuse for 15-20 minutes and filter. Wash your eyes and make compresses with the warm infusion.

✔ Sour cream mask with parsley greens

- 1 teaspoon of finely cut parsley greens

- 2 teaspoons of sour cream

Mix 1 teaspoon of finely cut parsley greens with 2 teaspoons of sour cream and put on your eyelids and skin under the eyes for 20 minutes. Then wash it off with cool water. This mask is recommended for edematous eyelids and exhausted eyes.

✔ Sour cream mask with tea

- 1 teaspoon of fatty sour cream

- 15 drops of castor or burdock oil

- Half a teaspoon of strong tea (black or green)

Add 15 drops of castor or burdock oil and half a teaspoon of strong tea (black or green) to 1 teaspoon of fatty sour cream. Stir well. Put this mixture on the wet skin of your eyelids with a cotton wool ball moistened with tea. Leave the mask for 20-30 minutes, then remove it with a wet cotton wool ball.

Lip care recipes

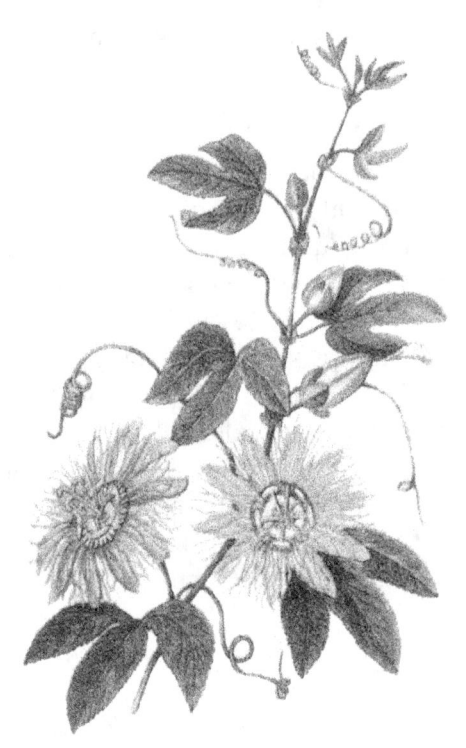

Lip care

The skin on the lips is as gentle and thin as the skin on eyelids. Sharply reacting to temperature drops, wind, frost and sun, it easily dries and chaps and small wrinkles appear above the lips. Daily care is necessary for lips to remain smooth and young for a long time. Much like the skin on your face, it is necessary to moisture, nourish and protect your lips. You should remove lipstick with the help of a cosmetic cream or milk. Also use regular masks with natural products, which should be applied no less than once a week to help keep your lips healthy and fresh.

There are many domestic means of lip care.

You can apply some carrot juice or a mix of it with honey (1:1) on your lips. It will prevent the occurrence of chapping and help to preserve natural color. Apply some honey to dry weather-beaten lips, and in few minutes wash it off with chamomile, calendula or eucalyptus tincture to quickly heal chapping. It is also useful to wipe your lips with a concentrated dogrose infusion every day. Sea-buckthorn oil is an effective means in the case of chapping along with calendula oil. Raw egg yolk, rendered goose fat, fresh butter, warm olive or castor oil, oil solutions with vitamins A and E and linseed extract (2 tablespoons per half a liter of water) all heal and soften dry lips very well. The use of lipstick is recommended when treating lips.

Vitamin and nourishing lip masks

These masks are particularly useful for chapped lips; lips with cracks, scratches and peeling skin. Apply and leave them for 10 minutes, then wash off with water and grease lips with vegetable oil. Such masks can also be applied as a preemptive measure once a week.

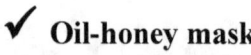 **Oil-honey mask**

- 1 teaspoon of olive oil

- 1 teaspoon of white (lime) honey

- 5 drops of carrot or beet juice

Mix 1 teaspoon of olive oil with 1 teaspoon of white (lime) honey and add 5 drops of carrot or beet juice. The mask heals and softens skin well, adding shine to the lips.

✔ Sour cream honey mask

- 1 teaspoon of white (lime) or May honey

- 1 teaspoon of fresh sour cream

Mix 1 teaspoon of white (lime) or May honey and fresh sour cream and apply this mixture to chapped lips.

✔ Creamy curd mask

- 1 teaspoon of curds

- 1 teaspoon of cream

Mix 1 teaspoon of curds with cream. This mask smoothes and softens lips.

✔ Curd-carrot mask

- 1 teaspoon of curds

- 1 teaspoon of carrot juice

Mix 1 teaspoon of curds with 1 teaspoon of carrot juice. This mask heals, moistens and nourishes lips.

✔ Apple mask

- Fresh apple pulp

- Butter

Mix the apple pulp and butter in equal parts. This mask softens the lips and heals cracks.

✔ Mask with kiwi and sea-buckthorn

- 1 teaspoon of kiwi pulp

- 8-10 drops of sea-buckthorn oil

Knead 1 teaspoon of kiwi pulp with 8-10 drops of sea-buckthorn oil. Sea-buckthorn and kiwi contain a lot of vitamin C and heal skin well.

Oils, ointments, creams for lip care

✔ Avocado oil

- 1 tablespoon of avocado oil

- 2 drops of rose oil

- 2 drops of sandalwood oil

Mix 1 tablespoon of avocado oil with 2 drops of rose oil and 2 drops of sandalwood oil. Grease dry lips with this mixture. This oil moistens and smoothes lips.

✔ Peach oil with honey

- 10 ml of peach oil

- 1 drop of lemon essential oil

- 1 drop of melissa essential oil

- 1 drop of chamomile essential oil

- Half a teaspoon of honey

Mix 10 ml of peach oil with lemon, melissa and chamomile essential oils (1 drop of each) and add half a teaspoon of honey. This oil heals cracks, making lips look fresh.

✔ Castor oil with honey

- 10 ml of castor oil
- 1 drop of lemon essential oil
- 1 drop of melissa essential oil
- 1 drop of chamomile essential oil
- Half a teaspoon of honey

Mix 10 ml of castor oil with the lemon, lavender and chamomile essential oils (1 drop of each) and add half a teaspoon of honey. This oil nourishes and moistens the lips, healing cracks.

✔ Ointment with rose petals

- 1 rose
- 1 tablespoon of unsalted pork fat

Crush fresh rose petals carefully and pound with 1 tablespoon of unsalted pork fat. Grease dry lips with cracks with this ointment.

✔ Honey ointment

- 1 teaspoon of honey
- Half a teaspoon of unsalted pork fat

Mix 1 teaspoon of honey with half a teaspoon of unsalted pork fat. This ointment softens lips and heals cracks.

✔ Lanolin cream

- 45 g of lanolin
- 1 teaspoon of castor oil
- 2–3 drops of rose oil

Melt 45 g of lanolin on a water bath, add 1 teaspoon of castor oil and stir, remove from the water bath and let it cool down. Then add 2-3 drops of rose oil and stir well again. Spread your chapped lips with this cream; it effectively softens and moistens.

✔ Cream with cocoa oil

- 7 g of cocoa oil

- 3 g of white beeswax

- 10 ml of castor, olive or peach oil

Melt 7 g of cocoa oil and 3 g of white beeswax on a water bath and add 10 ml of castor, olive or peach oil. This cream softens lips, eliminating dryness and peeling.

✔ Cream with cinquefoil rhizome

- 100 g of butter

- Half a tablespoon of dried cinquefoil rhizome powder

Melt 100g of butter, add half a tablespoon of dried cinquefoil rhizome powder and heat, stirring slowly, on a water bath for 10 minutes. Let it cool down and apply to your lips to heal cracks.

Frequently asked questions

✔ **How can I know if a skin care product is suitable for me?**

Before applying any skin care product (creams, masks, etc.) it is necessary to know your skin type. Before applying a mask for the first time it is necessary to carry out a "sensitivity test", otherwise even innocent wild strawberry pulp can cause negative effects for a person whose organism is sensitive to it.

✔ **How is it possible to determine one's type of skin?**

To determine your skin type you should carry out a skin type test.

✔ **In what conditions it is better to carry out skin care procedures?**

It is very important to find at least one and a half hours of full rest and peace when you are engaged with your appearance and skin care procedures. Absolute relaxation and a short nap during mask application is a guarantee of the benefit it will bring to you.

✔ **How do I correctly apply a skin care product to the face?**

All skin care procedures - cleansing of facial and neck skin, creams, powder, masks and their removal - are carried out strictly in accordance with skin lines.

✔**How should I apply creams and masks on the skin around the eyes correctly?**

You should apply creams (mask, lotions) on the skin around the eyes very carefully with your fingertips without stretching the skin.

✔ **What are the skin lines?**

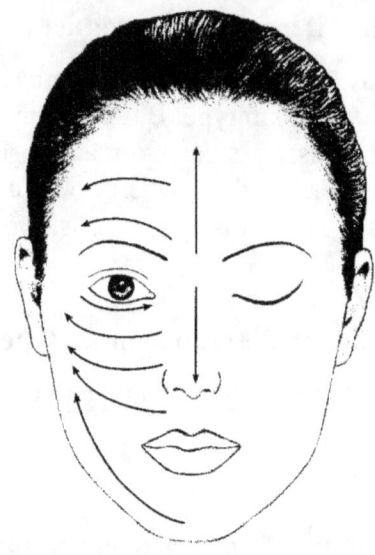

(Lines of the least stretching of face muscles)

Lines of the least stretched skin are referred to as skin lines. It is important that you accustom yourself with correct movements. Never treat your face and neck skin roughly or with force.

✔ **Where can I get ingredients for herbal/vegetable skin care products?**

Ingredients for herbal/vegetable skin care products are available in stores and at pharmacies. You can even prepare some ingredients for natural skin care products at home.

✔ **How much dried vegetable products and liquids are there in 1 tablespoon?**

In 1 tablespoon there are 3-5 g of dried ground leaves or flowers and grasses, 7-10 g of bark, rhizome and roots, 12 g of seeds, buds and fruits. Also in 1 tablespoon there are 15 ml of liquid while 1 teaspoon comprises 5 ml

✔ What tableware should be used for the preparation of vegetable skin care products (masks, creams, lotions, etc.)?

While preparing vegetable skin care products it is necessary to use glass, ceramic, wooden, enameled or plastic vessels.

✔ What is a water bath?

To construct a water bath pour some water into a bigger pot, then place a smaller pan inside it (the smaller one should contain the substance which is to be heated or boiled) and put on the heat. The small one should be hanging, i. e. not touching the bottom of the bigger pot, but floating in the water.

✔ How can I prepare rose water?

1. Add one handful of rose petals to 250 ml of boiling water and let it infuse in a closed vessel for 30 minutes. Filter it and use for cleansing of the face and neck. Rose water should be stored in glassware in a cool place.

2. Put petals of large fragrant dark red roses into a glass jar, fill it with 1 liter of boiling water and add 200 g of sugar. Let it infuse for two hours, stir and filter. Pour this rose water into a bottle and store in a dark cool place.

Warning:

Rose water possesses toning properties, so, you shouldn't apply it to places where blood vessels appear close to the skin.

✔ How can I prepare biostimulating aloe juice?

Cut off the bottom leaves of an aloe plant, wrap them in dark paper and keep in a refrigerator for 3 weeks at a temperature of 2-4 °C. As a result new substances (biogenic stimulators) are formed in these leaves. Then wash the leaves with cold water, chop, add water in a 1:3 proportion and keep in a dark, cool place for 1.5 hours. After that wring the juice out and filter it.

✔ **How can I prepare a tincture or extract?**

Pour some water in a vessel with crushed vegetative ingredients in accordance with the recipe. If the proportion of raw material and water is not specified in the recipe, it is usually 1:10, i.e. 1 part of raw material to 10 parts of water. You can make more strong extractions (in 1,5-2 times) for external use.

To prepare a tincture you should place raw material in a porcelain, enameled or glass vessel, fill it with boiled water, close with a cover and leave to infuse for the time determined by the recipe.

If the process of infusion takes a lot of time, cover a vessel with a towel. But it is better to prepare tinctures in the following way: put raw material into an enameled pot with a cover, pour some water of room temperature (about 20 °C) in it and heat it on a water bath without boiling. Do not put the pot directly on the flame. You should heat it on a water bath for 15 minutes.

Use the same method for the preparation of extracts, but raw material is boiled for 30 minutes (or prepared in the way specified in the recipe). The heating time is increased by 10 minutes if more water is used (1 liter and more).

After heating the solution is cooled at room temperature: tinctures for no less than 10 minutes, extracts for 45 (in a warm place). It is then filtered through a cloth or two layers of gauze; the rest is wrung out and the portion of liquid received is also filtered. If it is necessary add some boiled water.

In some cases tinctures are prepared without heating by infusing raw material for a certain period of time (from 4 to 12 hours) in cold water at room temperature. Tinctures or extracts prepared from plants containing tannins (oak bark, tutsan herb, etc.) should be filtered immediately after heating as they quickly grow turbid and spoil when cooled.

Tinctures from seeds and roots are prepared by adding hot water in certain proportions. Upon infusion termination they are shaken and filtered.

Use fresh tinctures and extracts as they lose their curative properties in storage. Keep them in a refrigerator for no longer than two days.

✔ **What juices are better to use for the preparation of vegetative skin care products?**

Vegetative skin care product preparation requires only freshly squeezed juices as they do not contain preservatives.

✔ **Why are self-made creams so effective?**

The main aspect of such creams is freshness. The cream is prepared from fresh natural products, without preservatives and harmful chemical additives. The fat base of such a cream consists of beeswax, lanolin, cocoa oil, vegetable oil or animal fats. Medicinal herbs, fruit, vegetable and berry juices, honey and dairy products that are included in its structure nourish and rejuvenate skin.

It is necessary to remember that natural components of home-made creams spoil rather quickly, therefore these creams can be kept in a refrigerator but not for a long time: from several days to about two weeks.

Skin type test

Read the 50 statements in our test carefully. Mark everything you think can be attributed to you.

1	My skin shrinks unpleasantly after each cleansing.	A
2	Red spots appear rather often on my face and neck.	F
3	I cannot wash my face with soap.	F
4	Skin on my face is very dry.	F
5	I have to cream my skin at least three times a day in order to make it soft and look smooth.	A
6	After almost each application of a new cosmetic product pink or red spots appear on my skin.	F
7	I can use any cosmetics without any unpleasant consequences.	B
8	My skin always seems oily.	C
9	If I use powder, my face already seems "spotty" after an hour.	C
10	I have to carry a powder box with me because my nose is constantly shining.	D
11	Skin around the eyes becomes flabby.	E
12	My face shines as if I have just applied cream to it.	C
13	I have consulted a dermatologist because of the hyperirritability of my skin.	F
14	I am inclined to allergic reactions.	F
15	Many wrinkles have appeared around my eyes.	E
16	My nose and forehead shine on my face.	D
17	Noticeable wrinkles have appeared on my skin.	E
18	My skin absorbs cream like a sponge.	E
19	I think that powder dries my skin.	A
20	After a walk my skin gains a beautiful pink color.	B
21	When I come from outdoors my skin has shrunk.	A
22	I feel relief as soon as I cream my skin.	A
23	My skin sunburns very quickly.	F
24	My complexion is more likely to be white.	F
25	I have a healthy complexion almost all the year round.	B
26	I suffer from sleeplessness; sometimes I can't fall asleep for hours.	E

27	I think that pores on my skin are rather large.	C
28	I frequently suffer from acne and pimples.	C
29	My skin is matte and it never shines.	A
30	Pimples appear rather often on my nose-forehead area.	D
31	It seems to me that I have "strong" skin.	B
32	In the center of my face pores are visible more distinctly than on my cheeks.	D
33	An especially big portion of nourishing cream is needed for my skin after visiting the pool, otherwise it feels shrunk for several hours.	A
34	I take diuretic agents regularly.	A
35	I am over 35 years of age.	E
36	I visit the solarium regularly and frequently sunbathe in the summer.	A
37	My skin often starts to itch if I stay in a hot heated room for a long time.	F
38	I would like my skin to be more elastic.	E
39	Freckles appear very quickly on my skin.	E
40	If direct sunbeams reach my skin, it burns immediately.	F
41	My sunburn is rather even.	B
42	My skin seems very thin and transparent.	E
43	I have been washing myself with water and soap only for many years.	B
44	When I pluck my eyebrows, red spots remain on my skin for an hour after that.	F
45	If any important event is approaching, I usually gain pimples on my face or herpes on my lips.	F
46	Bad sleep is immediately reflected on my appearance.	E
47	I can't do without conditioner at work.	A
48	My skin is oilier in the summer than in the winter.	D
49	Until now a universal cream has been quite enough for me.	B
50	If I use a light day cream, my cheeks become too dry.	D

The most frequently occurring marked letter will point out your type of skin. If two or more letters occur an equal number of times, your skin is of combined type. Every fifth woman has a combined type of skin (for example, dry and sensitive simultaneously). In a cosmetic sense, it isn't a complicated problem though.

Does the letter "**B**" prevail in your marked answers?
- You have NORMAL skin.

Does the letter "**C**" prevail in your marked answers?
- You have OILY skin.

Does the letter "**A**" prevail in your marked answers?
- You have DRY skin.

Does the letter "**D**" prevail in your marked answers?
- You have COMBINED skin.

Does the letter "**F**" prevail in your marked answers?
- You have PROBLEM-PRONE skin.

Does the letter "**E**" prevail in your marked answers?
- You have MATURE skin.